CW01017620

VEGAN COOKBOOK

BREAKFAST EDITION

Plant-Based Breakfast Recipes with Easy Instructions

DANA TAYLOR

© Copyright 2021 - All rights reserved.

The content contained within this book may not be reproduced, duplicated or transmitted without direct written permission from the author or the publisher.

Under no circumstances will any blame or legal responsibility be held against the publisher, or author, for any damages, reparation, or monetary loss due to the information contained within this book. Either directly or indirectly.

Legal Notice:

This book is copyright protected. This book is only for personal use. You cannot amend, distribute, sell, use, quote or paraphrase any part, or the content within this book, without the consent of the author or publisher.

Disclaimer Notice:

Please note the information contained within this document is for educational and entertainment purposes only. All effort has been executed to present accurate, up to date, and reliable, complete information. No warranties of any kind are declared or implied. Readers acknowledge that the author is not engaging in the rendering of legal, financial, medical or professional advice. The content within this book has been derived from various sources. Please consult a licensed professional before attempting any techniques outlined in this book.

By reading this document, the reader agrees that under no circumstances is the author responsible for any losses, direct or indirect, which are incurred as a result of the use of information contained within this document, including, but not limited to, errors, omissions, or inaccuracies.

TABLE OF CONTENTS

VEGAN PEANUT BUTTER AND JELLY OVERNIGHT OATS

Vegan peanut butter and jelly overnight oats, a delicious and healthy breakfast or snack to eat on the go or to make the day before to save some time every morning.

MAKES 2 SERVING/ TOTAL TIME 10 MINUTE

INGREDIENTS

3/4 cups rolled oats (90 g), gluten-free if needed

3/4 cup unsweetened soy milk (200 ml)

1 tbsp maple or agave syrup

2 tbsp peanut or almond butter

2 tbsp raspberry jam

2 bananas, chopped

Chopped peanuts (optional)

METHOD

STEP 1

There are several ways you can make this recipe. You can add all the ingredients to a jar, stir, cover and keep in the fridge overnight (or for at least 4 hours), or add all the ingredients except the bananas and add them the next morning (bananas are best when fresh and this way we prevent oxidation), or add the rolled oats and milk and add the rest of the ingredients the next morning. I prefer option number 3, but it's up to you. If you chose option number 1, you'll save some extra time every morning.

Stir the overnight oats before eating and add more milk if needed.

NUTRITION VALUE

441 Energy, 12.1g fat, 2.4g saturated fat, 7.7g fiber, 12.4g protein, 76.4g carbs.

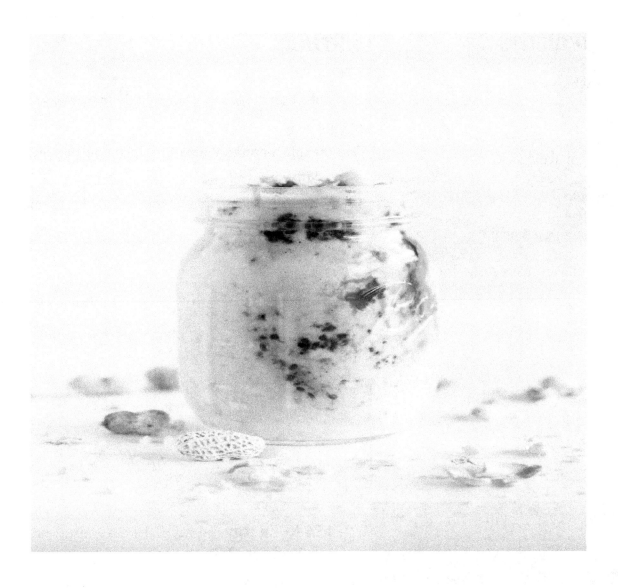

TROPICAL FRUIT SALAD

This tropical fruit salad is a delicious, simple and healthy recipe, made with fresh fruit, lime or lemon juice and maple or agave syrup.

MAKES 2 SERVING/ TOTAL TIME 10 MINUTE

INGREDIENTS

12 strawberries

2 kiwis

1/2 dragon fruit, see notes

1/2 mango

1 tbsp lime or lemon juice

2 tsp maple or agave syrup (optional)

METHOD

STEP 1

Peel and chop the fruits. Then add them to a large mixing bowl.

Add the lime or lemon juice and the maple or agave syrup. Stir until well combined.

Best when fresh, keep leftovers in a sealed container in the fridge for 1 to 2 days.

NUTRITION VALUE

154 KJ Energy, 1g fat, 0.1g saturated fat, 5.1g fiber, 2.3g protein, 37.5g carbs.

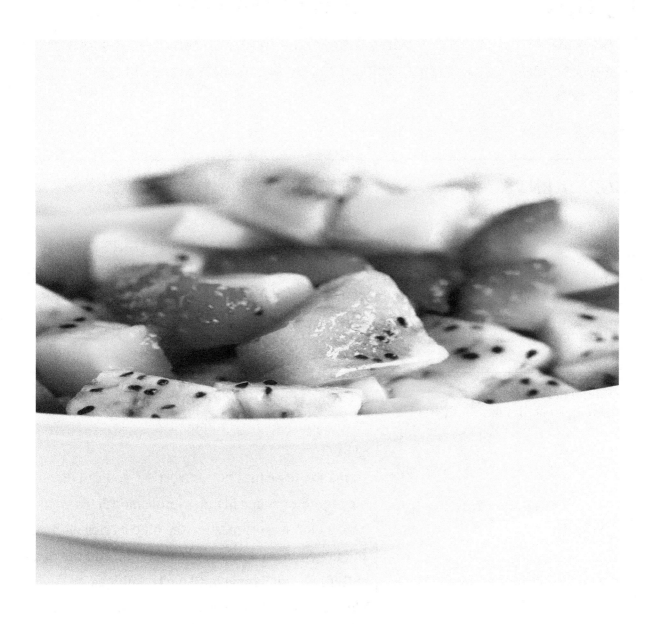

VEGAN GLUTEN FREE LEMON BLUEBERRY CAKE (10 MINUTES)

Vegan gluten-free lemon blueberry cake, made in just 10 minutes! It's low in fat and the perfect dessert or breakfast recipe if you want something sweet and easy to make.

MAKES 2 SERVING/ TOTAL TIME 10 MINUTE

INGREDIENTS

for the cake:

- 1/2 banana
- 4 tbsp full-fat coconut milk
- 4 tbsp cane, coconut or brown sugar
- 4 tbsp flour, we used buckwheat flour
- 1 tbsp lemon juice
- 1/2 tsp baking soda
- 1/4 cup fresh blueberries (40 g) + some extra blueberries as topping (optional)
- The zest of half a lemon (optional)

for the peanut butter frosting (optional):

- 3 tbsp full-fat coconut milk
- 2 tbsp peanut butter
- 2 tbsp fresh blueberries

METHOD

STEP 1

Add the half banana to a mixing bowl and mash it with a fork. Then add the rest of the ingredients and stir until well combined. You can also blend all the ingredients in a blender to get a smoother texture, but it's not necessary.

Add the blueberries and lemon zest and stir again.

Place the bowl in a side of the microwave, not in the center and cook for 4 minutes.

STEP 2

To make the peanut butter frosting, you can blend all the ingredients in a blender until smooth. As we didn't have a blender, we mashed the blueberries with a fork and mixed them with the coconut milk and the peanut butter in a small bowl until well combined.

We didn't add all the frosting to the cake for the pictures, but we ate it all with the cake. Besides, we also topped the cake with some extra blueberries.

NUTRITION VALUE

1190 KJ Energy, 8.7g fat, 1.9g saturated fat, 13.6g fiber, 11.3g protein, 32.2g carbs.

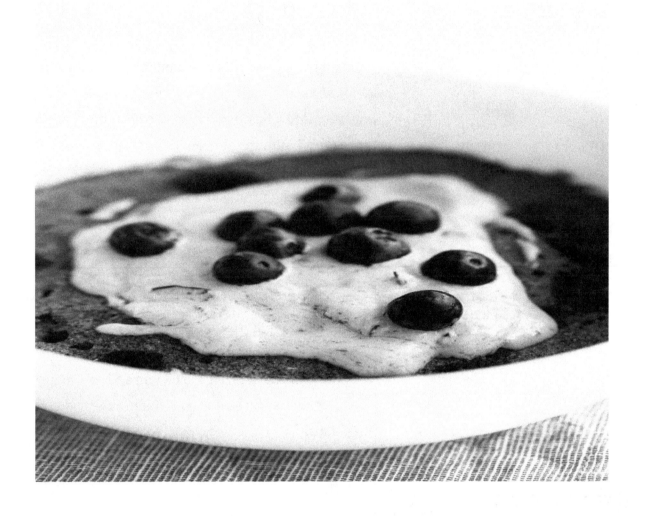

SIMPLE VEGAN FRENCH TOAST

8-ingredient vegan French toast! This recipe makes a delicious breakfast or brunch that everyone loves in less than 30 minutes.

MAKES 6 SERVING/ TOTAL TIME 25 MINUTE

INGREDIENTS

1 and 1/2 cups plant milk of your choice (375 ml), we used oat milk

2 tbsp flaxseeds

2 tbsp maple or agave syrup

1/2 tsp vanilla extract (optional)

1/4 tsp ground cinnamon

1/8 tsp sea salt

6–8 slices (1-inch-thick or 2.5 cm) bread, preferably day old (see notes)

Coconut oil (optional)

METHOD

STEP 1

Add all the ingredients to a blender (except the bread and the coconut oil) and blend until smooth. Pour the mixture into a baking dish or a shallow bowl and let stand for 5 minutes at room temperature.

Place each slice of bread into the mixture, allowing the bread to soak in some of it on both sides.

STEP 2

Heat some coconut oil in a griddle or a hot skillet, and place the bread slices onto the griddle/hot skillet until browned on one side, then flip and brown the other side (about 5 minutes for each side).

Serve with your favorite toppings. We added some maple syrup, berries, chia seed jam and soy yogurt. Keep leftovers in a sealed container in the fridge for 3 to 4 days.

NUTRITION VALUE

176 Energy, 4.1g fat, 1.7g saturated fat, 2.2g fiber, 3.1g protein, 31.6g carbs.

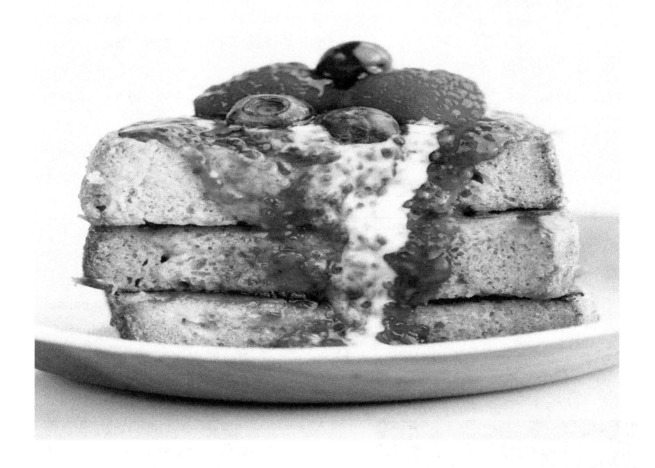

HOW TO MAKE CHIA SEED JAM

It requires 10 minutes and 5 ingredients. Feel free to use any fresh or frozen fruit or any sweetener you have on hand.

MAKES 1 SERVING/ TOTAL TIME 10 MINUTE

INGREDIENTS

2 cups fresh raspberries (250 g) or any other fresh or frozen fruit

1 tbsp water

1 tbsp lemon juice

3 tbsp chia seeds

3 tbsp maple or agave syrup

METHOD

STEP 1

Add raspberries and water to a saucepan and cook over medium-hight heat for about 2 minutes, stirring occasionally.

Use a fork or potato masher to mash the raspberries to your desired consistency.

Add lemon juice, chia seeds and syrup. Stir and cook for 2 to 3 minutes. Then taste and add more syrup if needed.

STEP 2

Remove from heat and let cool for 5 minutes (it will thicken considerably as it cools).

Stir the jam one more time and serve immediately, or keep it in a sealed container in the fridge for up to 1 week.

NUTRITION VALUE	27 KJ Energy, 0.7g fat, 0.1g saturated fat, 1.7g fiber, 0.1g protein, 5.2g carbs.

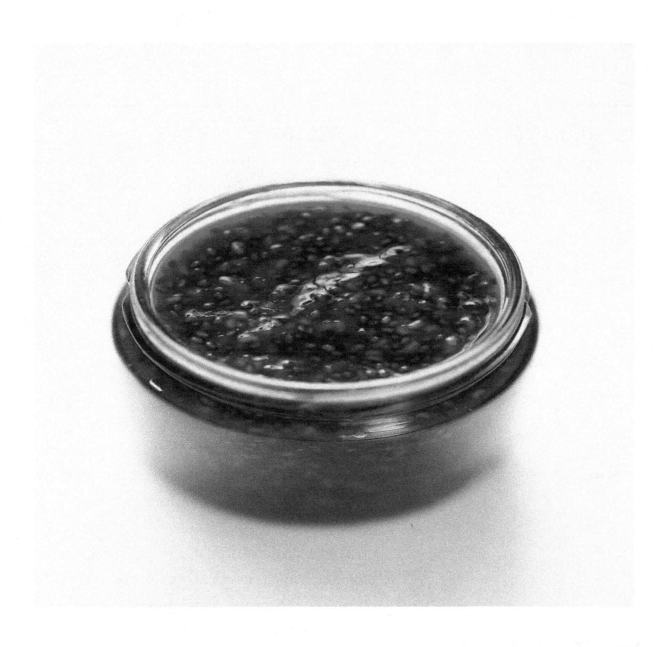

VEGAN BAKED PUMPKIN DONUTS (GLUTEN-FREE)

Vegan baked pumpkin donuts made in just 25 minutes. They're gluten-free, low in fat and so delicious. It's a super healthy breakfast recipe!

MAKES 6 SERVING/ TOTAL TIME 25 MINUTE

INGREDIENTS

1/2 cup and 2 tbsp oat flour (80 g)

1/2 cup and 2 tbsp light buckwheat flour (75 g)

1/4 cup cane, coconut or brown sugar (50 g)

1 tsp pumpkin pie spice

1/2 tsp baking soda

1/2 cup full fat coconut milk (125 ml)

1/4 cup pumpkin puree (65 g)

1 and 1/2 tsp apple cider vinegar

METHOD

STEP 1

Preheat the oven to 400ºF or 200ºC.

Combine the oat flour, buckwheat flour, sugar, pumpkin pie spice and baking soda in a large mixing bowl.

Add the coconut milk, pumpkin puree and vinegar to the bowl and mix until well combined.

Feel free to grease the donut pan with some coconut oil if you want. I don't do this, but it's up to you.

Fill each pan cavity approximately 3/4 full.

STEP 2

Bake for about 15 minutes or until golden brown.

Remove from the oven and allow the donuts to cool for at least 10 minutes before removing them from the donut pan. Then place on a wire rack to cool completely.

When the donuts were cold, we covered them with some cinnamon sugar, but it's optional. We blended 2 tbsp cane sugar with 1/2 tsp ground cinnamon in a blender, but you can also mix them in a bowl.

NUTRITION VALUE

150 KJ Energy, 5.9g fat, 4.3g saturated fat, 2.2g fiber, 3.2g protein, 22.3g carbs.

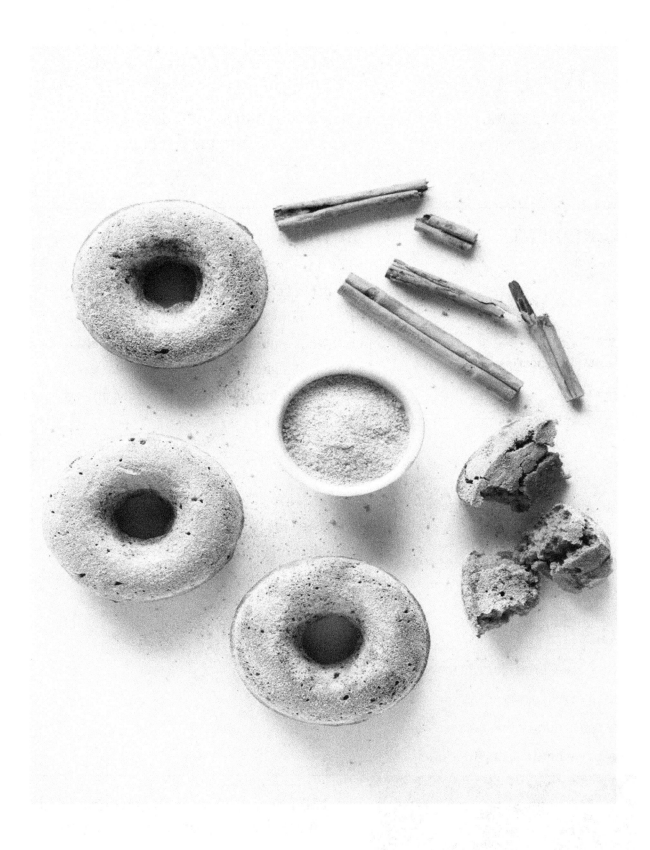

VEGAN GLUTEN-FREE BERRY CRISP (LOW-FAT)

This vegan gluten-free berry crisp is a delicious and low-fat dessert or breakfast recipe. Feel free to use any fresh or frozen fruit you like.

MAKES 2 SERVING/ TOTAL TIME 35 MINUTE

INGREDIENTS

For the filling:

1 cup raspberries (120 g)

1/2 cup blackberries (75 g)

1/2 cup blueberries (70 g)

2 tbsp flour,

2 tbsp cane, brown or coconut sugar

1 tbsp lemon juice

1 tbsp water

1/4 tsp ground cinnamon

For the topping:

1/2 cup oats, use gf if needed (50 g)

1/4 cup flour,

1/4 cup chopped raw and unsalted almonds (30 g)

2 tbsp cane, brown or coconut sugar

1 tbsp maple or agave syrup

1/2 tsp ground cinnamon

Vegan cashew frosting (optional)

METHOD

STEP 1

Preheat the oven to 350ºF or 180ºC.

Add the filling ingredients to a mixing bowl and mix until well combined using a spoon or your hands.

Add the filling to a baking dish .

Add the topping ingredients to a bowl and mix until well combined.

STEP 2

Add to the top of the filling in an even layer.

Bake for 20 to 25 minutes or until the top is golden brown and the fruit is bubbling. The time may vary depending on the oven.

Let the crisp cool for at least 10 minutes before serving. You can eat it hot or cold.

NUTRITION VALUE

160 Energy, 3.6g fat, 0.3g saturated fat, 4.7g fiber, 2.8g protein, 31.5g carbs.

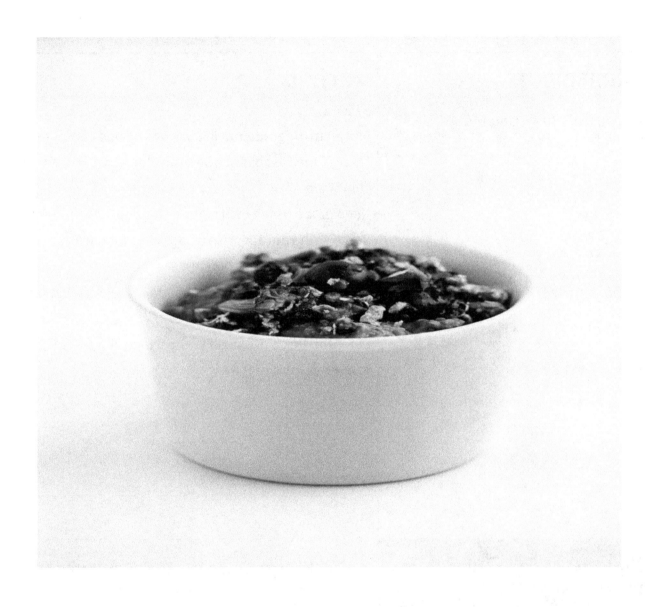

VEGAN BIRCHER MUESLI

This vegan Bircher muesli is a delicious, healthy, quick and easy breakfast recipe, but you can also have it as a snack or dessert.

MAKES 2 SERVING/ TOTAL TIME 5 MINUTE

INGREDIENTS

1 cup oats (100 g), gluten-free if needed

1 and 1/2 cups plant milk of your choice (375 ml), we used full fat coconut milk

1 tbsp chia seeds

2 tbsp Sultana raisins

2 tbsp pumpkin seeds

1 tbsp agave syrup

Fresh raspberries and blueberries

METHOD

STEP 1

Mix all the ingredients in a jar or a sealed container (except the raspberries and the blueberries) until well combined.

Keep in the fridge overnight or for at least 4 hours.

Serve with your favorite fruits. We added fresh raspberries and blueberries.

If it's too dry for you, you can add more milk just after serving.

Store the Bircher muesli in the fridge in a sealed container for 2 to 3 days.

NUTRITION VALUE

396 Energy, 23.7g fat, 16.8g saturated fat, 8.1g fiber, 10.1g protein, 40.6g carbs.

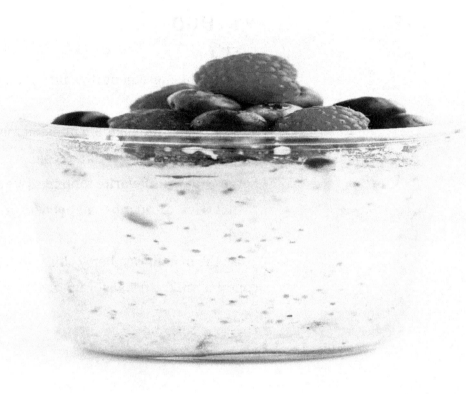

INSTANT RASPBERRY CHIA PUDDING

This super creamy raspberry chia pudding is made with just 4 ingredients and as it's instant, you can eat it immediately, so you don't have to wait.

MAKES 4 SERVING/ TOTAL TIME 5 MINUTE

INGREDIENTS

1 cup fresh raspberries (150 g)

3/4 cup plant milk of your choice (190 ml), we used unsweetened almond milk

1/2 cup chia seeds (85 g)

3 tbsp maple or agave syrup

METHOD

STEP 1

Place all the ingredients in a blender and blend until smooth.

You can serve the pudding immediately, but we prefer to keep it in the fridge until is cold.

Serve with your favorite toppings (we added mashed raspberries, cacao nibs, chopped walnuts and sesame seeds).

Store the instant raspberry chia pudding in a sealed container in the fridge for up to 4 days.

NUTRITION VALUE

183 Energy, 9.2g fat, 1.1g saturated fat, 11.2g fiber, 5.1g protein, 21.9g carbs.

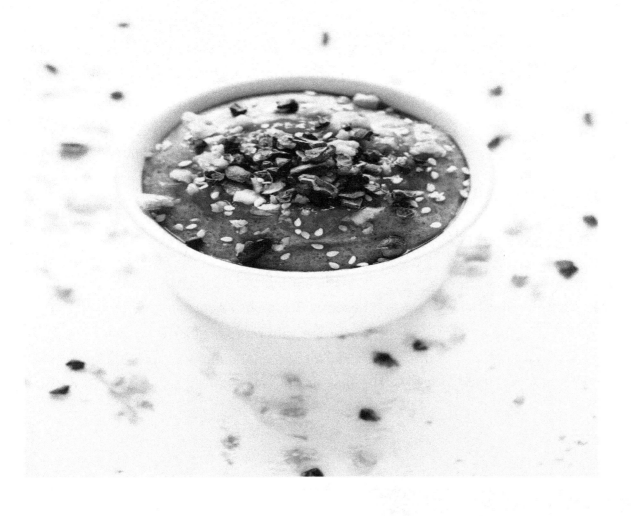

VEGAN LEMON CAKE (GLUTEN FREE)

This vegan gluten-free lemon cake is low in fat, oil and yeast free and is made with unrefined ingredients. It's so healthy and delicious.

MAKES 8 SERVING/ TOTAL TIME 40 MINUTE

INGREDIENTS

1 cup brown rice flour (140 g)

1 1/4 cup oat flour* (140 g)

1/2 cup cane sugar (100 g)

2 tsp baking soda

3 flax eggs

1 cup coconut milk (250 ml)

1/2 cup lemon juice (125 ml)

1 tbsp lemon zest

Vegan cashew frosting to taste (optional)

We added some almonds, blueberries and more lemon zest on top (optional)

METHOD

STEP 1

Preheat the oven to 400ºF or 200ºC.

Mix the dry ingredients in a large mixing bowl (the brown rice flour, oat flour, sugar and baking soda).

STEP 2

Make the flax eggs.

Add the flax eggs, coconut milk, lemon juice and lemon zest to the bowl and mix until well combined.

Grease the cake pan with some oil (coconut oil is my favorite one). If you use a non-stick pan, you can omit this step. We usually place a sheet of parchment paper on the bottom of the cake pan to avoid using oil. We used an 8 2/3 " or 22 cm pan in diameter.

Pour the batter into the pan.

Bake for about 30 minutes or until it's fully cooked.

Remove the cake from the oven and let it cool down completely.

NUTRITION VALUE

266 Energy, 9.7g fat, 5.9g saturated fat, 3.1g fiber, 5.2g protein, 41.6g carbs.

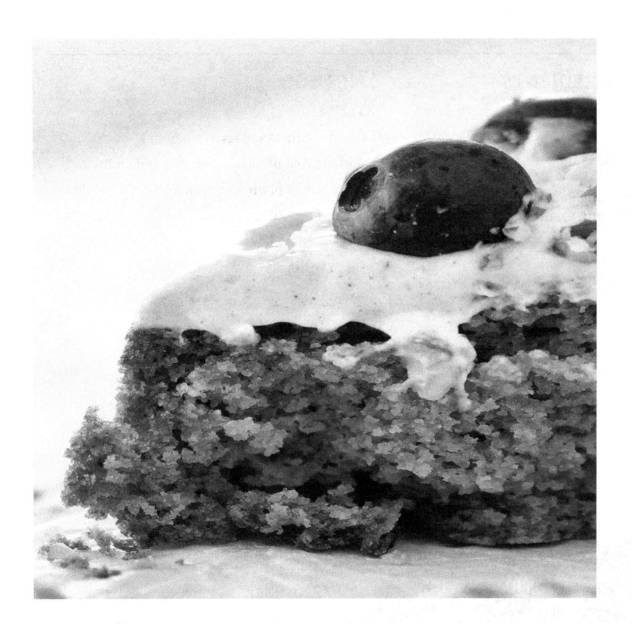

3-INGREDIENT VEGAN GF PANCAKES

These vegan pancakes are a great healthy breakfast, whether you like sweet or savory.

MAKES 6 SERVING/ TOTAL TIME 20 MINUTE

INGREDIENTS

1 banana

1 cup instant oats (100 g)

3/4 cup plant milk of your choice (185 ml), we used oat milk

METHOD

STEP 1

Grind the instant oats in a blender.

Add the rest of the ingredients and blend until smooth.

Place ¼ cup of the batter in a non-stick skillet (or a lightly greased skillet) and cook for about two minutes for each side.

Serve with your favorite toppings.

NUTRITION VALUE

98 Energy, 1.5g fat, 0.2g saturated fat, 2.5g fiber, 2.9g protein, 18.9g carbs.

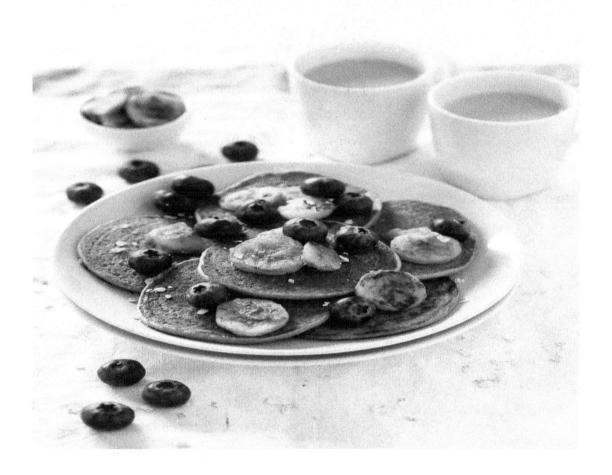

VEGAN APPLE AND BLACKBERRY CRUMBLE (FAT FREE)

This vegan apple and blackberry crumble tastes great and is a super healthy dessert or breakfast. We prefer to eat it cold with some plant milk.

MAKES 4 SERVING/ TOTAL TIME 35 MINUTE

INGREDIENTS

For the fruit layer:

2 peeled and diced apples*

2 cups fresh or frozen blackberries (300 g)

4 tbsp brown or coconut sugar**

1 tsp cinnamon powder

1 tbsp lemon juice

2 tbsp water

For the topping:

1 1/3 cup rolled or instant oats (160 g)

1 tsp ground cinnamon

3 tbsp agave or maple syrup

3 tbsp brown or coconut sugar

METHOD

STEP 1

Place all the ingredients for the fruit layer in a saucepan and cook over high heat. Bring it to a boil and then cook over medium-high heat for about 10 minutes or until the fruit is cooked. Pour the fruit layer into a baking dish and set aside.

STEP 2

Preheat the oven to 355ºF or 180ºC.

In the meanwhile, we're going to make the topping.

Place the oats and the ground cinnamon in a mixing bowl and heat the syrup and the sugar in a saucepan over high heat until the sugar is melted. Stir frequently. Pour this mixture into the bowl and mix until well combined.

Place the topping onto the fruit layer.

Bake for about 10 to 20 minutes or until golden brown. And the crumble is ready to eat!

NUTRITION VALUE

164 Energy, 1.1g fat, 0.2g saturated fat, 5.3g fiber, 2g protein, 39.1g carbs.

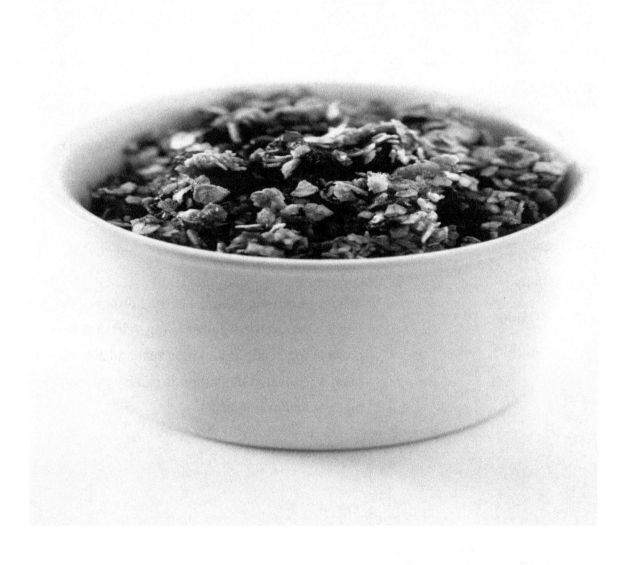

MANGO CHIA PUDDING

This mango chia pudding is a super healthy and quick breakfast meal, but you can also eat it as a snack or even as a dessert. It's perfect to eat on the go!

MAKES 2 SERVING/ TOTAL TIME 15 MINUTE

INGREDIENTS

1 cup almond milk (250 ml)*

4 tbsp chia seeds

2 tbsp maple syrup

1 chopped mango

Lime zest (optional)

Almond flakes (optional)

METHOD

STEP 1

Combine the milk, seeds and syrup in a bowl or a sealed container and let stand for 15 minutes at room temperature. Stir, cover and let stand in the fridge overnight or for at least 4 hours.

STEP 2

Place some mango chunks at the bottom of the glasses, bowls or containers you're using. Add the chia mixture, more mango chunks and lime zest and almond flakes to taste. We toasted the almonds in a frying pan without oil for a few minutes.

NUTRITION VALUE

144 Energy, 4.7g fat, 0.7g saturated fat, 6.2g fiber, 3g protein, 24.7g carbs.

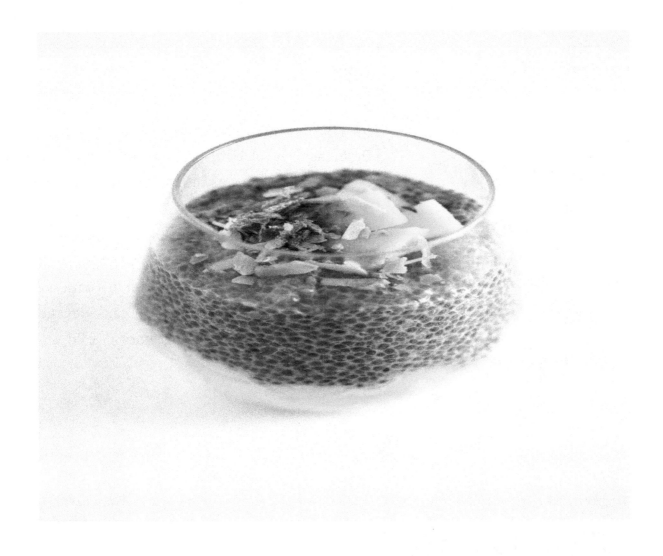

SIMPLE VEGAN CASHEW YOGURT

Making non-dairy yogurt at home is so easy, besides, it's healthier and tastes so good! We used unsalted raw cashews to make this delicious vegan yogurt.

MAKES 6 SERVING/ TOTAL TIME 10 MINUTE

INGREDIENTS

2 2/3 cups unsalted raw cashews (400 g)

1 1/2 cup water (375 ml)

4 tbsp lemon juice

1/4 tsp sea salt

3 probiotic supplements

METHOD

STEP 1

Soak the cashews overnight.

Drain them and place them in a blender with the rest of the ingredients (except the supplements) and blend until smooth.

Place the yogurt in a bowl, add the 3 supplements (we need the powder, so empty the capsules). Mix well. Cover with a cheesecloth and let it sit in a dark, cool room for at least 12 hours. Then you can enjoy the yogurt or keeping it in the fridge until it's cold.

NUTRITION VALUE

258 KJ Energy, 19.8g fat, 3.5g saturated fat, 1.5g fiber, 8.3g protein, 14.1g carbs.

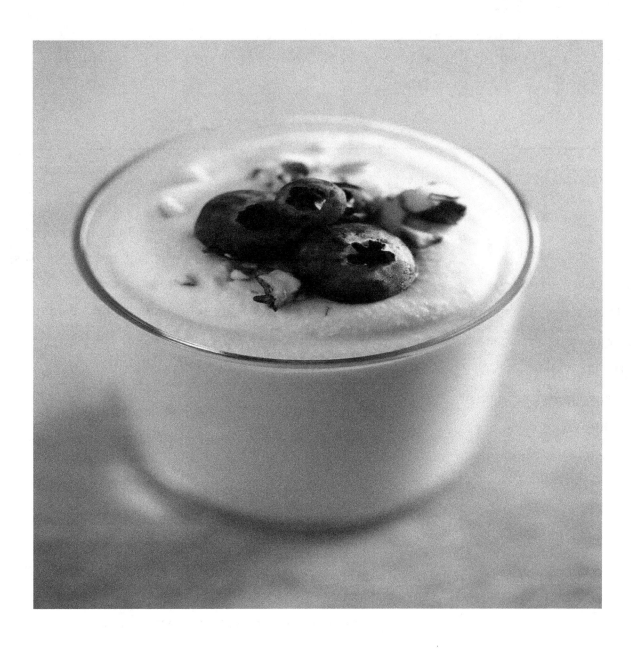

POMEGRANATE GLAZED BRUSSELS SPROUTS

These Pomegranate Glazed Brussels Sprouts are made in the oven and toss with a 2-ingredient Pomegranate glazed (pomegranate juice and soy sauce). It's easy, quick and very delicious.

MAKES 4 SERVING/ TOTAL TIME 35 MINUTE

INGREDIENTS

4 cups brussels sprouts - bottom part of the brussels sprouts removed, and chop them in half.

2 tablespoons olive oil

1 teaspoon garlic - minced

Salt and pepper to taste

FOR THE POMEGRANATE GLAZE:

½ cup pomegranate juice

2 tablespoons soy sauce

1 garlic clove - minced

METHOD

STEP 1

Pre-heat the oven to 400F degrees. In a big bowl, add brussels sprouts, olive oil, garlic, salt and pepper. Toss until everything is evenly coated.

Spread the brussels sprouts mixture onto a baking sheet in an even layer. The cut-side of the brussels should be touching the baking sheet.

STEP 2

You should bake them for about 25-20 minutes or until the brussels sprouts are golden brown on the edges. The baking time will depend on the size of your brussels sprouts and the power of your oven.

Meanwhile, in a small saucepan over medium-high heat pour all the ingredients for the pomegranate glaze. Bring to a boil for 5 - 8 minutes, and stir well until thick and syrupy.

Top with the pomegranate glaze. Enjoy!

NUTRITION VALUE

141 KJ Energy, 7.3g fat, 1.1g saturated fat, 3.4g fiber, 3.5g protein, 18.1g carbs.

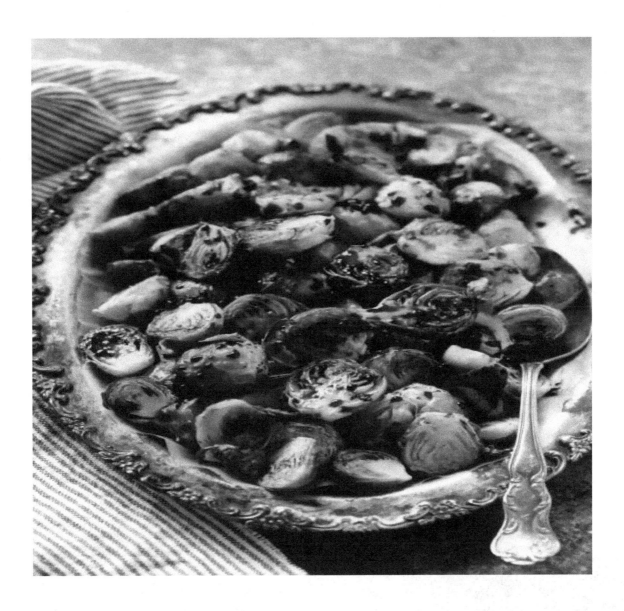

5-INGREDIENT OATMEAL COOKIES

These 5-ingredient oatmeal cookies are super chewy and not as crunchy as others, but they're the healthiest cookies you can make and taste amazing.

MAKES 20 SERVING/ TOTAL TIME 30 MINUTE

INGREDIENTS

1 banana

½ cup applesauce (160 g)

4 tbsp agave syrup

2 cups rolled oats (240 g)

½ cup raisins (80 g)

METHOD

STEP 1

Preheat the oven to 390ºF or 200ºC. Mash the banana in a bowl, then add the applesauce and agave syrup and stir. Add the rolled oats and raisins and stir until well combined.

STEP 2

Scoop the dough (about 1.5 tablespoons each) onto a baking sheet with baking parchment. Press down on the dough mounds with your hands or a tablespoon to slightly flatten.

Bake the cookies until golden brown (for about 15 to 20 minutes).

Remove and let set for about 5 minutes on the pan.

Then transfer the cookies to a cooling rack until they're cool.

NUTRITION VALUE

62 Energy, 0.6g fat, 0.1g saturated fat, 1.2g fiber, 1.3g protein, 13.5g carbs.

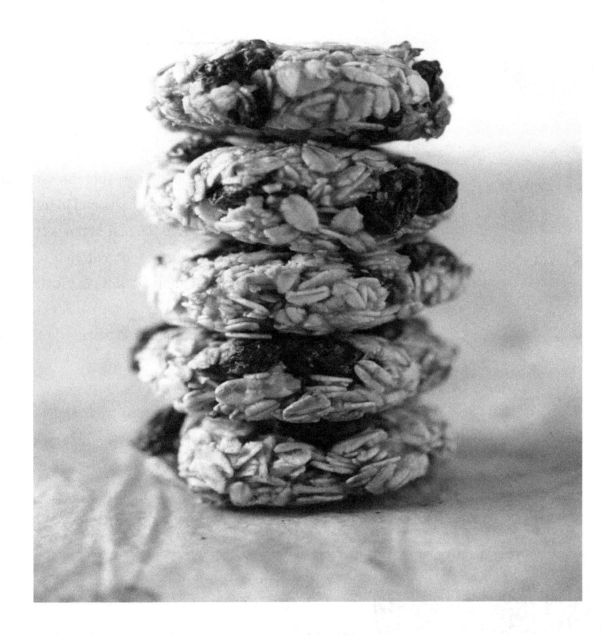

SIMPLE VEGAN DEHYDRATED COOKIES

Dehydrating food only minimally affects its nutritional value, which is great! You're going to love these simple vegan dehydrated cookies.

MAKES 30 SERVING/ TOTAL TIME 20 MINUTE

INGREDIENTS

2 apples

4 tbsp flax seeds

1 tsp ground cinnamon

1/2 cup almonds (80 g)

1/2 cup dates (100 g)

4 cup oats (480 g)

METHOD

STEP 1

Place all the ingredients in a food processor excluding the oats and blend for a few seconds. Place the cookie dough in a big mixing bowl, add the rest of the oats and mix with your hands. Add 2 cups of oats and blend again until well combined. Add the rest of the oats (another 2 cups) and mix using a spoon or your hands. If the dough is too wet, add more oats, if it's too dry, add some water.

Make the cookies using your hands. We made 1/4-inch cookies (1/2 cm).

STEP 2

Place the cookies into the dehydrator trays and dehydrate to 45ºC or 113ºF for about 4 hours for one side and another 2 hours for the other side. The time may vary depending on your dehydrator or the ingredients you're using.

NUTRITION VALUE

72 Energy, 1.89g fat, 0.2g saturated fat, 2.2g fiber, 2g protein, 12.3g carbs.

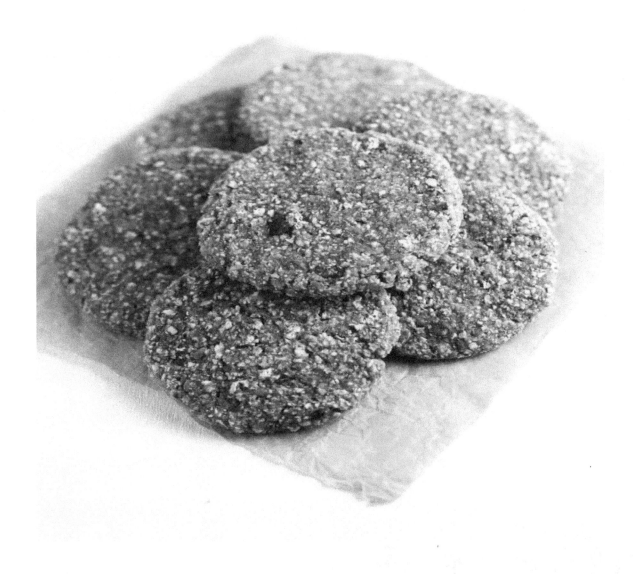

OIL FREE PANCAKES (VEGAN + GLUTEN FREE)

These oil-free pancakes are vegan an also gluten-free. Best healthy pancakes ever!

MAKES 7 SERVING/ TOTAL TIME 25 MINUTE

INGREDIENTS

1/2 cup oat flour (60 g)

1/2 cup buckwheat flour (70 g)

1 tsp baking powder

1/2 tsp ground cinnamon

3/4 cup oat milk (185 ml)

1 banana

1 tbsp almond butter

1 tbsp maple syrup

Toppings: blueberry jam and fresh figs

METHOD

STEP 1

Mix dry ingredients in a bowl (oat flour, buckwheat flour, baking powder and cinnamon).

Place the rest of the ingredients in a blender and blend until smooth.

Combine dry and wet ingredients in a bowl and stir with a spoon.

STEP 2

Place ¼ cup of batter in a non-stick skillet (or a lightly greased skillet) and cook for about two minutes for each side.

Serve with your favorite toppings.

NUTRITION VALUE

106 Energy, 2.3g fat, 0.3g saturated fat, 2.5g fiber, 3.1g protein, 19.8g carbs.

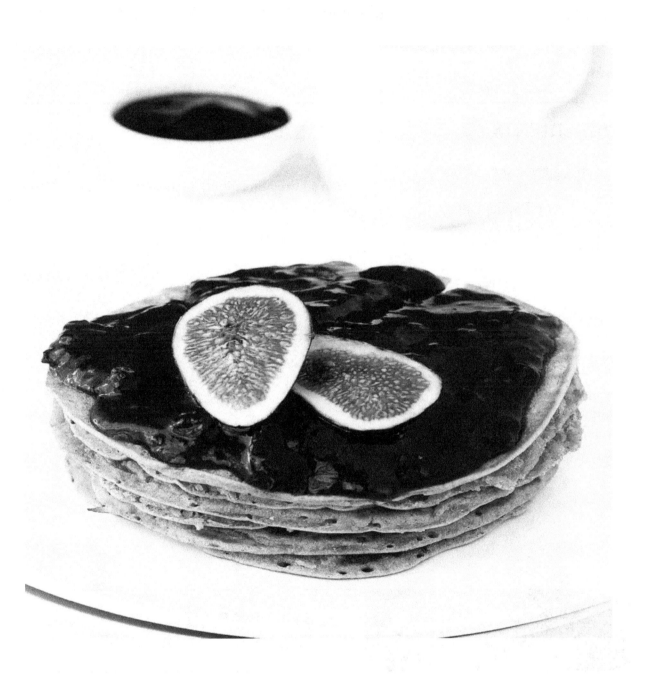

BLUEBERRY SMOOTHIE BOWL

Breakfast is my favorite meal and sometimes I make a huge smoothie bowl, I love it!

MAKES 2 SERVING/ TOTAL TIME 10 MINUTE

INGREDIENTS

2 frozen + 2 regular bananas

1/2 cup almond milk (125 ml)

4 Medjool dates or 8 Deglet Nour

1 cup frozen blueberries (155 g)

1/4 cup rolled oats (40 g)

1 tbsp Chia seeds

Toppings: sliced banana, shredded coconut, fresh strawberries, chopped raw and unsalted almonds and rolled oats

METHOD

STEP 1

Place all the ingredients in a blender and blend until smooth.

Add your favorite toppings.

NUTRITION VALUE

556 Energy, 18.3g fat, 13.3g saturated fat, 15.3g fiber, 7.8g protein, 102.5g carbs.

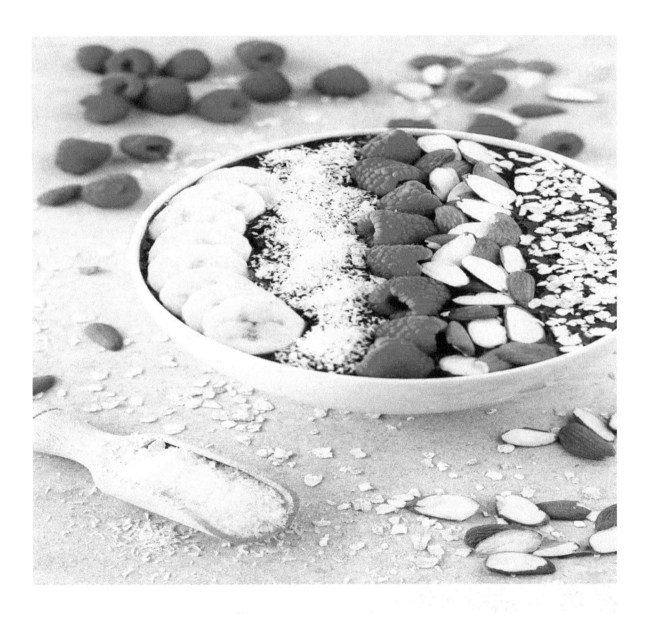

OIL FREE GRANOLA

Granola is super easy to make and it lasts up to 3 weeks. This oil free granola is so delicious, you won't notice any difference!

MAKES 10 SERVING/ TOTAL TIME 35 MINUTE

INGREDIENTS

2 cups rolled oats (200 g)

1 cup chopped almonds (160 g)

1 cup chopped dates (170 g)

½ cup Goji berries (60 g)

½ cup sunflower seeds (70 g)

1 tbsp ground cinnamon

½ cup water (125 g)

1 tsp vanilla extract (optional)

⅔ cup maple syrup (215 g)

METHOD

STEP 1

Preheat the oven to 320ºF or 160ºC.

Mix the dry ingredients in a big bowl (rolled oats, chopped almonds, chopped dates, Goji berries, sunflower seeds and ground cinnamon).

In a saucepan, heat the wet ingredients (water, vanilla extract and maple syrup) for about 2 minutes. Pour over the dry ingredients and mix well.

STEP 2

Spread the granola onto a baking tray and bake for 25 minutes or until golden brown, stirring every 10 minutes to get a more crumbly granola.

Remove from the oven and allow the granola to cool completely. Store in an airtight container at room temperature for up to 3 weeks.

NUTRITION VALUE

262 Energy, 7.5g fat, 0.7g saturated fat, 5.5g fiber, 5.3g protein, 46.8g carbs.

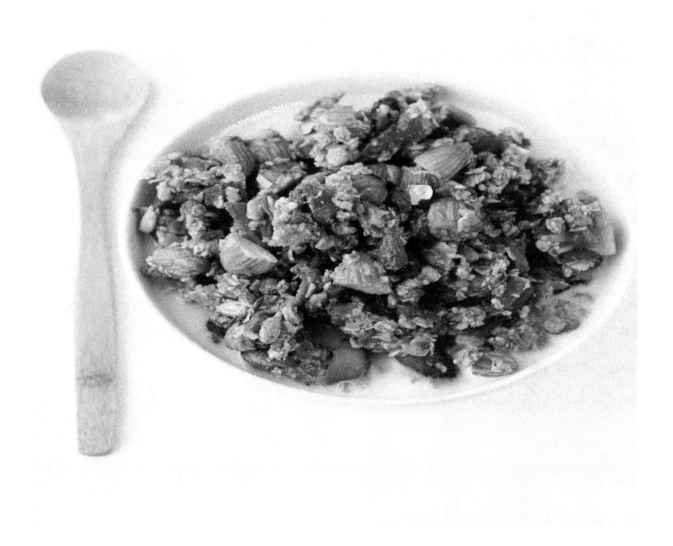

PUMPKIN CHOCOLATE CHIP PANCAKES

These pumpkin chocolate chip pancakes are vegan and gluten-free. They are the perfect pancakes and also lighter and healthier than traditional pancakes.

MAKES 9 SERVING/ TOTAL TIME 30 MINUTE

INGREDIENTS

1 cup chopped pumpkin or pumpkin puree (150g)

1 cup rice flour (150 grams)

1 cup oat flour (120 grams)

2 tsp baking powder

1 1/4 cups rice milk (300 milliliters)

2 tbsp maple syrup

1 tbsp coconut oil

1 tsp cinnamon

1/8 tsp ground ginger

1/8 tsp nutmeg

1 clove

1/2 cup chocolate chips (90 grams)

METHOD

STEP 1

Mix dry ingredients in a bowl (rice flour, oat flour, baking powder, cinnamon, ginger and nutmeg). You can make your own oat flour grinding oats in a food processor or a grinder.

Mix wet ingredients in another bowl (milk, maple syrup and oil).

STEP 2

Add the chopped pumpkin (or the pumpkin puree) and the wet ingredients in a blender and blend. Add the dry ingredients and blend again.

Pour the batter in a bowl, add the chocolate chips and stir with a spoon.

Place ¼ cup of batter in a hot pan lightly greased and cook for about two minutes for each side or until golden brown. You will know they are ready to flip when bubbles form on top and the edges appear dry.

NUTRITION VALUE

216 Energy, 6g fat, 3.7g saturated fat, 2.9g fiber, 4.7g protein, 36.7 carbs.

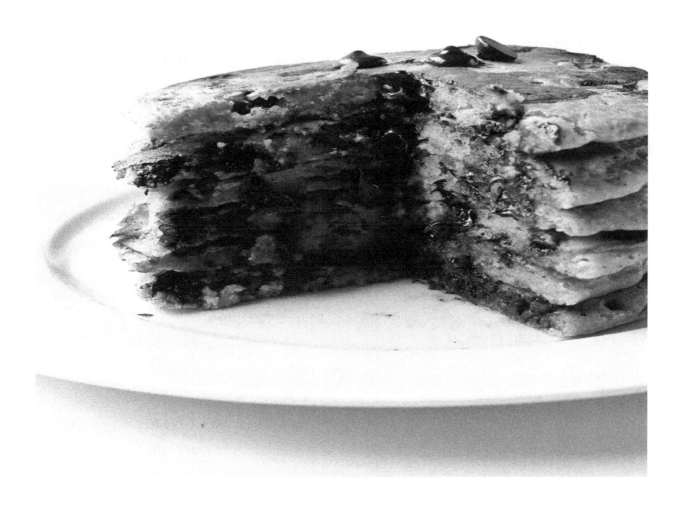

PEANUT BUTTER GRANOLA

Breakfast is the most important meal of the day, but you can eat healthy and also enjoy your breakfast. Try this peanut butter granola, it's delicious!

MAKES 8 SERVING/ TOTAL TIME 30 MINUTE

INGREDIENTS

For the granola:

2 cups oats (200g)

1/2 cup dried cranberries (75 g)

1 cup hazelnuts (150g)

2 tbsp water

1 tsp vanilla extract (optional)

2 tbsp coconut oil

1/3 cup maple syrup (100 g)

1/3 cup peanut butter (90 g)

For the jam:

1 cup blueberries (150 g)

2 tbsp water

The juice of a quarter of a lemon

6 tbsp coconut sugar

0.05 oz agar (1 g) (optional)

METHOD

STEP 1

Preheat the oven to 320 ºF or 160 ºC.

Place in a bowl the oats, dried cranberries and hazelnuts. Pour into a saucepan the water, vanilla extract, coconut oil, maple syrup and peanut butter, stir and cook over medium heat for 2 or 3 minutes Combine dry and wet ingredients in the bowl and stir with a wooden spoon until all ingredients are totally mixed.

STEP 2

Place the granola on a baking sheet (with baking paper) and bake for 25 minutes.

Remove from the oven and allow the granola to cool completely. Place in a glass container and it should keep for a few weeks.

To make the jam you only have to place in a saucepan the blueberries, water, lemon juice and sugar and cook over medium heat for 30 minutes. You can add agar to thicken, but it's optional.

NUTRITION VALUE

346 Energy, 5.3g fat, 5.3g saturated fat, 5.5g fiber, 8.9g protein, 31.9g carbs.

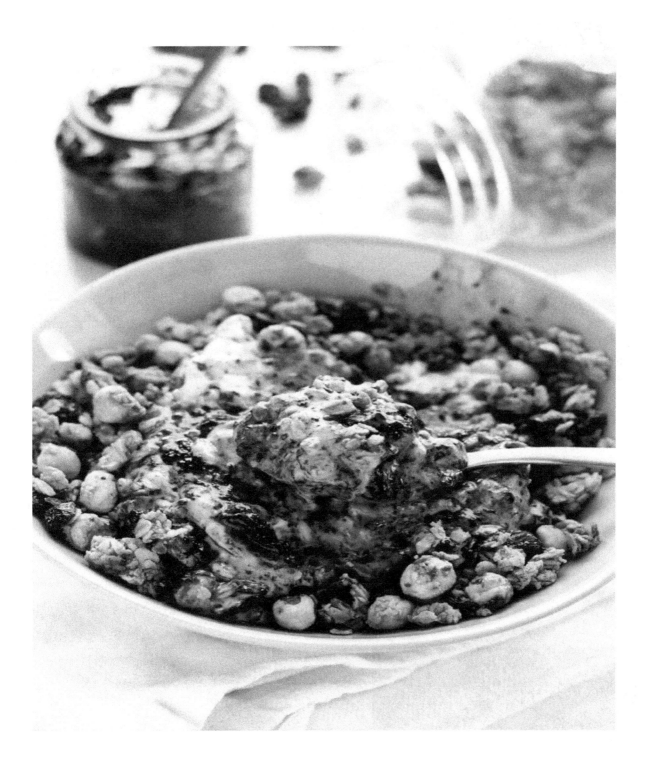

SOY YOGURT

To make homemade soy yogurt you're going to need only two ingredients: soy milk and a starter. So simple and cheap.

MAKES 8 SERVING/ TOTAL TIME 10 MINUTE

INGREDIENTS

4 cups soy milk (1 liter)

1 teaspoon agar powder

1/2 cup soy yogurt (125 grams) or yogurt starter powder (the amount may vary, follow the package instructions)

METHOD

STEP 1

Preheat the oven at 50º C or 120º F.

Pour the soy milk in a saucepan, add the agar, stir and heat the mixture to 90º C or 195º F, but be careful because it shouldn't boil. You can use a thermometer, but it's not necessary.

Pour the mixture in a bowl and let it cool to 40 or 50ºC (105º F or 120º F). If you don't have a thermometer, you can put your finger in the mixture and when it's hot but not burn it's ready.

STEP 2

Add the starter (soy yogurt or yogurt starter powder), stir and pour the mixture into glass jars or containers. Turn off the oven, place the glass jars or containers (without lids) inside and let stand for at least 8 hours. You mustn't open the oven during this process.

NUTRITION VALUE

61 Energy, 2.9g fat, 0.3g saturated fat, 1.4g fiber, 5.6g protein, 3.4g carbs.

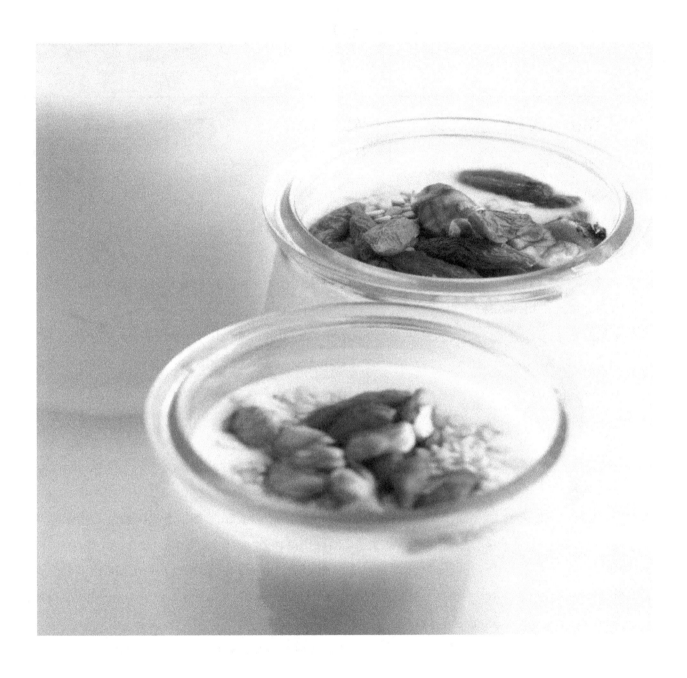

KALE, BLACK BEAN & AVOCADO BURRITO BOWL

This recipe is both gluten free and vegan.

MAKES 4 SERVING/ TOTAL TIME 50 MINUTE

INGREDIENTS

1 cup brown rice, rinsed

¼ teaspoon salt

Lime marinated kale

1 bunch curly kale,

¼ cup lime juice

2 tablespoons olive oil

½ jalapeño, seeded

½ teaspoon cumin

¼ teaspoon salt

1 avocado, pitted and sliced into big chunks

½ cup mild salsa Verde

Seasoned black beans

2 cans black beans, rinsed and drained

1 shallot, finely chopped

3 cloves garlic, pressed or minced

¼ teaspoon chili powder

METHOD

STEP 1

Bring a big pot of water to a boil, dump in rinsed brown rice and boil, uncovered, for 30 minutes. Turn off the heat, drain the rice and return it to the pot. Cover and let the rice steam in the pot for 10 minutes, then fluff the rice with a fork and season with ¼ teaspoon salt, Whisk together the lime juice, olive oil, chopped jalapeño, cumin and salt. Toss the chopped kale with the lime marinade in a mixing bowl.

STEP 2

Combine the avocado chunks, salsa Verde, cilantro and lime juice and blend well.

Warm the beans: In a saucepan, warm 1 tablespoon olive oil over medium-low heat. Sauté the shallot and garlic until fragrant, then add the beans, chili powder and cayenne pepper. Cook until the beans are warmed through and softened, stirring often, about 5 to 7 minutes. If the beans seem dry at any point, mix in a little splash of water.

Garnish with chopped cherry tomatoes.

NUTRITION VALUE

1190 KJ Energy, 8.7g fat, 1.9g saturated fat, 13.6g fiber, 11.3g protein, 32.2g carbs.

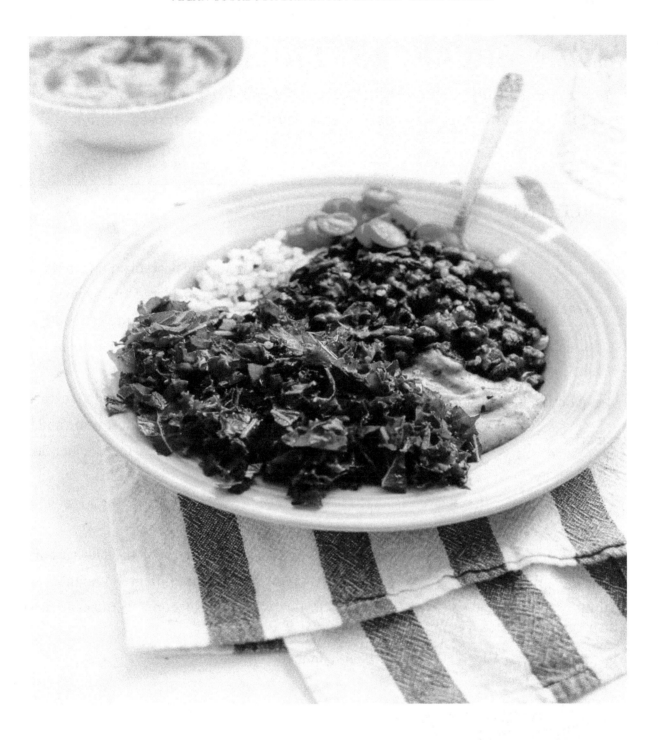

VEGAN BREAKFAST SAUSAGE

Vegan breakfast sausage made with textured vegetable protein, flour, vegetable stock and tons of herbs and spices. It tastes like the real thing!

MAKES 10 SERVING/ TOTAL TIME 30 MINUTE

INGREDIENTS

1 cup textured vegetable protein (80 g)

1 cup vegetable stock

1 and 1/4 cups brown rice flour (175 g)

1/4 cup nutritional yeast (4 tbsp)

2 tsp dried sage

2 tsp dried thyme

2 tsp garlic powder

1/2 tsp paprika

1/8 tsp ground black pepper

2 tbsp tamari or soy sauce

1 tbsp maple syrup

2 flax eggs

METHOD

STEP 1

Add the textured vegetable protein and the hot vegetable stock or water to a large mixing bowl. Stir, cover and allow to sit for 5-10 minutes to absorb.

Mix the dry ingredients in another large mixing bowl until well combined.

Add the rest of the ingredients (rehydrated textured vegetable protein, tamari or soy sauce, syrup and flax eggs) to the bowl you have the dry ingredients. Stir until well combined.

STEP 2

Make 10-12 patties with your hands.

Heat some oil in a skillet and cook the sausages until golden brown for both sides (about 3-4 minutes each side). If you don't eat oil, just omit it. You can also cook the sausages in a Griddler.

Serve immediately.

NUTRITION VALUE

106 Energy, 1.5g fat, 3.3g fiber, 6.2g protein, 16g carbs.

56

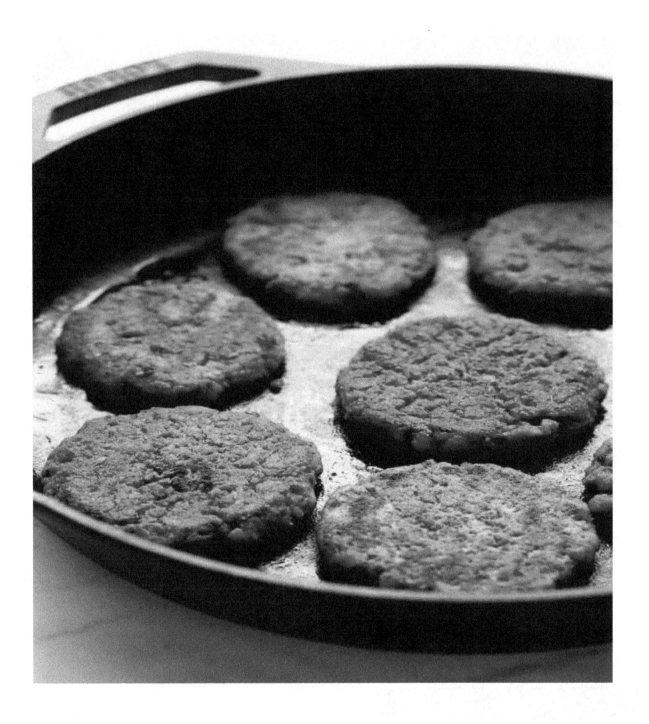

VEGAN PEANUT BUTTER AND JELLY OVERNIGHT OATS

Vegan peanut butter and jelly overnight oats, a delicious and healthy breakfast or snack to eat on the go or to make the day before to save some time every morning.

MAKES 2 SERVING/ TOTAL TIME 10 MINUTE

INGREDIENTS

3/4 cups rolled oats (90 g), gluten-free if needed

3/4 cup unsweetened soy milk (200 ml)

1 tbsp maple or agave syrup

2 tbsp peanut or almond butter

2 tbsp raspberry jam

2 bananas, chopped

Chopped peanuts (optional)

METHOD
STEP 1
There are several ways you can make this recipe. You can add all the ingredients to a jar, stir, cover and keep in the fridge overnight (or for at least 4 hours), or add all the ingredients except the bananas and add them the next morning (bananas are best when fresh and this way we prevent oxidation), or add the rolled oats and milk and add the rest of the ingredients the next morning. I prefer option number 3, but it's up to you. If you chose option number 1, you'll save some extra time every morning.

Stir the overnight oats before eating and add more milk if needed.

You can keep it covered in the fridge for 3 to 4 days. It's also a great breakfast or snack to eat on the go.

NUTRITION VALUE

441 Energy, 12.1g fat, 2.4g saturated fat, 7.7g fiber, 12.4g protein, 76.4g carbs.

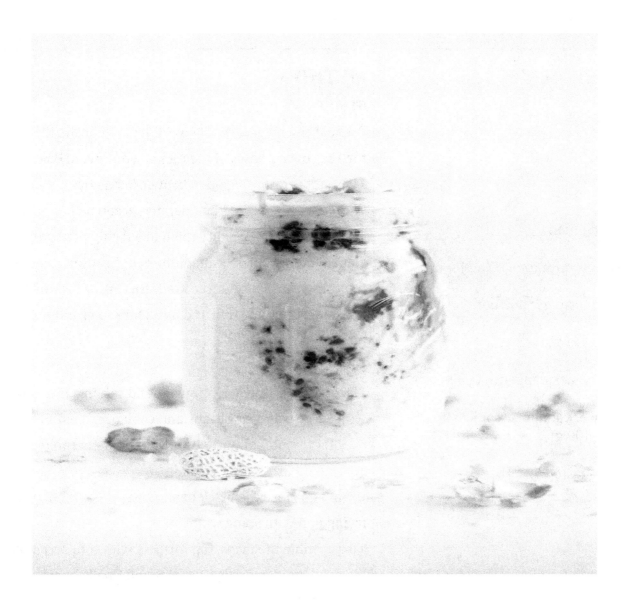

VEGAN BREAKFAST TACOS

These 30-minute vegan tacos are perfect for breakfast. You can also eat them for lunch or dinner, they're so delicious, healthy and satisfying.

MAKES 6 SERVING/ TOTAL TIME 30 MINUTE

INGREDIENTS

6 whole wheat or corn tortillas

1/2 red bell pepper

1/2 green bell pepper

1/2 red onion

10 ounces firm tofu (275 g)

1/4 tsp turmeric powder

1/4 tsp sea salt

Ground black pepper to taste

15 ounces canned or cooked black beans (400 g)

Salsa to taste

1 avocado

METHOD

STEP 1

Preheat the oven to 400ºF or 200ºC and drape the tortillas over 2 rows of the rack of your oven. Bake for 10 minutes or until golden brown. Set aside.

Chop the veggies (red bell pepper, green bell pepper and red onion) and sauté them in a frying pan with some water or oil over medium-high heat for about 5 minutes or until they're cooked, stirring occasionally. Set aside. Chop the tofu and use a fork to crumble it into bite-sized pieces.

STEP 2

Place the tofu, turmeric powder and salt in a frying pan with some water or oil, stir and cook over medium-high heat for about 5 minutes or until the tofu is cooked, stirring occasionally. Set aside.

Drain and rinse the black beans and reheat them in the frying pan with some water.

To assemble the tacos, top tortillas with tofu scramble, black beans, some salsa, veggies and finally some avocado slices.

NUTRITION VALUE	435 Energy, 14.4g fat, 2.6g saturated fat, 11.5g fiber, 19.3g protein, 60g carbs.

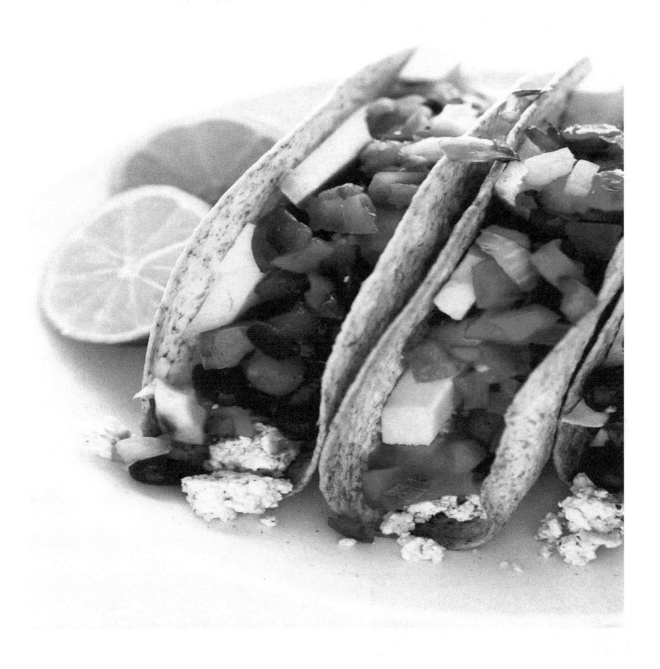

BREAKFAST POTATOES

Breakfast potatoes, made with 7 ingredients in just 30 minutes. They're so crispy on the outside, creamy on the inside, and super easy to make.

MAKES 2 SERVING/ TOTAL TIME 30 MINUTE

INGREDIENTS

1-pound potatoes (450 g), peeled if desired and diced

1–2 tbsp extra-virgin olive oil

2 tsp Italian seasoning or any other dried herb

1/2 tsp salt

1/2 tsp garlic powder

1/2 tsp paprika

1/8 tsp ground black pepper

METHOD

STEP 1

Preheat the oven to 400ºF or 200ºC.

Add all the ingredients to a large mixing bowl and mix until well combined (I prefer to use my hands).

Place the potatoes onto a lined baking sheet and bake for 20-30 minutes or until soft and golden brown

Serve immediately with sauces like vegan mayo, healthy ketchup, barbecue sauce, vegan aioli, and vegan sour cream. You could also eat them as part of a vegan brunch with fresh fruit, vegan butter, and homemade jelly toasts, tofu scramble, and natural orange juice or coffee. Another option is serving your breakfast potatoes with any vegan meat substitute like seitan or tempeh bacon.

NUTRITION VALUE

219 Energy, 7.3g fat, 1.1g saturated fat, 5.7g fiber, 4g protein, 36.2g carbs.

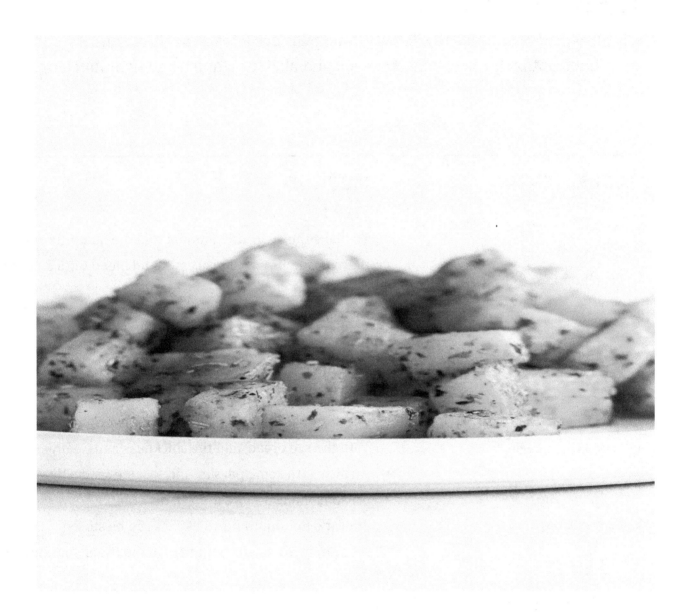

AVOCADO HUMMUS TOASTS WITH CHICKPEAS

These avocado hummus toasts with chickpeas are a tasty, healthy and nutritious option for breakfast or snack and also for a quick and light lunch or dinner.

MAKES 4 SERVING/ TOTAL TIME 20 MINUTE

INGREDIENTS

4 bread slices, we used German rye bread

1/3 cup hummus (80 g)

1/4 avocado

7 oz canned or cooked chickpeas (200 g)

1 tsp cumin powder

1/2 tsp garlic powder

1/2 tsp paprika

1/4 tsp salt

1/8 tsp ground black pepper

2 tbsp extra-virgin olive oil or tahini

Chopped fresh parsley and sesame seeds for garnish (optional)

METHOD

STEP 1

To make the avocado hummus, add the hummus and the avocado in a food processor and blend until smooth. Set aside.

STEP 2

Place the chickpeas in a mixing bowl with the rest of the ingredients You can eat them cold or hot. We prefer to cook them in a frying pan until they're warm.

To assemble the toasts spread some avocado hummus onto the rye bread, add the chickpeas and finally garnish with some parsley and sesame seeds. Heat the bread if you want (we didn't).

Avocado hummus and chickpeas can be stored separately in sealed containers in the fridge for about 4 days.

NUTRITION VALUE	140 Energy, 7.4g fat, 1g saturated fat, 4.9g fiber, 5.1g protein, 14.8g carbs.

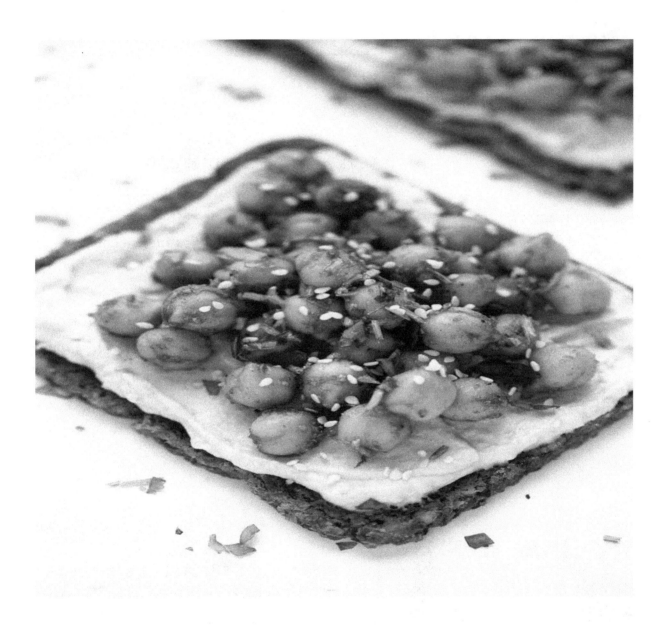

TOMATO AVOCADO SALAD (OIL-FREE)

A simple tomato avocado salad, made in less than 10 minutes with just 4 ingredients and our oil-free tahini salad dressing.

MAKES 4 SERVING/ TOTAL TIME 10 MINUTE

INGREDIENTS

1 cup corn kernels, frozen or canned (140 g)

4 salad tomatoes

2 medium avocados

1 red onion

Tahini salad dressing

METHOD

STEP 1

If you use frozen corn kernels, cook them according to package directions and then drain them. If you use canned corn kernels, drain and wash them. Set aside.

STEP 2

Chop the tomatoes, avocados and red onion.

Mix all the ingredients in a large mixing bowl (corn, tomatoes, avocados, red onion and tahini salad dressing) until well combined. Serve immediately.

Best when fresh, keep leftovers in a sealed container in the fridge for 1 to 2 days (dressing separate from the salad).

NUTRITION VALUE

386 Energy, 24.3g fat, 5.4g saturated fat, 11.5g fiber, 8.2g protein, 21.5g carbs.

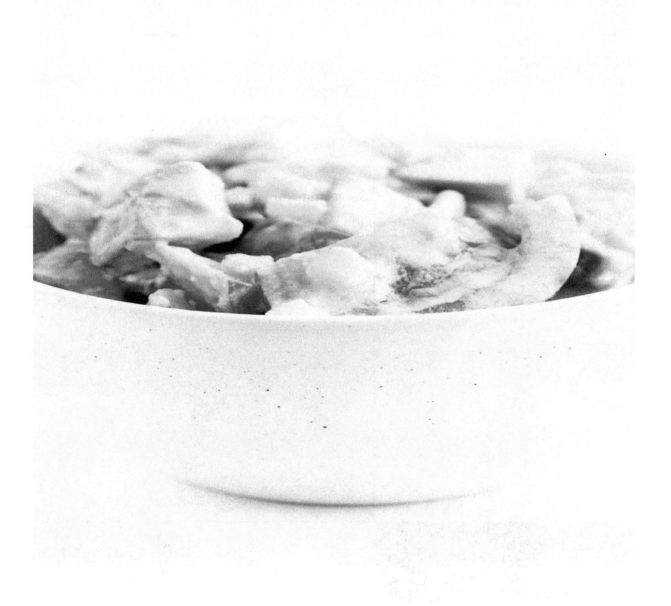

BANANA BLUEBERRY SMOOTHIE

This banana blueberry smoothie is the perfect breakfast smoothie, but you can also have it for lunch or dinner.

MAKES 1 SERVING/ TOTAL TIME 5 MINUTE

INGREDIENTS

1 banana

1 cup blueberries (150 g)

1 cup spinach (30 g)

1/4 cup oats (25 g)

1 cup plant milk of your choice or water*

METHOD

STEP 1

Place the banana, blueberries, spinach, oats and milk in a blender and blend until smooth.

Serve and your smoothie is ready to drink. Feel free to add any natural sweetener, like dates or coconut sugar.

NUTRITION VALUE

385 Energy, 6.1g fat, 0.9g saturated fat, 11.3g fiber, 8.4g protein, 79.1g carbs.

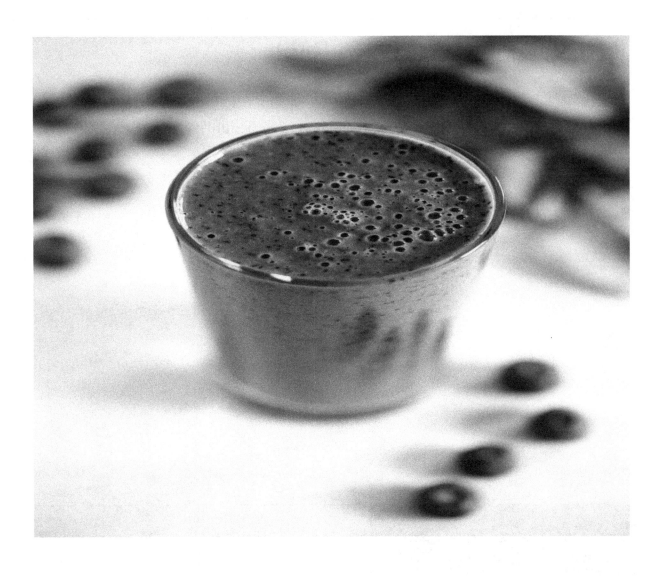

BUTTER PEANUT BANANA TOAST

To make these peanut butters, banana, coconut toast you just need 4 ingredients and 10 minutes.

MAKES 1 SERVING/ TOTAL TIME 10 MINUTE

INGREDIENTS

Coconut flakes

Bread slices, see notes

Peanut or almond butter

Banana, sliced

METHOD

STEP 1

Add the coconut flakes to a skillet and cook over medium-high heat until golden brown, stirring frequently (optional).

Toast the bread slices in a skillet, toaster or oven (optional).

Spread the peanut or almond butter onto the bread slices while they're still hot (this way it will be easier and they will taste better).

Add the banana slices and top with some toasted coconut flakes.

Best with fresh, you can also eat them on the go.

NUTRITION VALUE

222 Energy, 9.7g fat, 2.5g saturated fat, 4.5g fiber, 8.3g protein, 28.4g carbs.

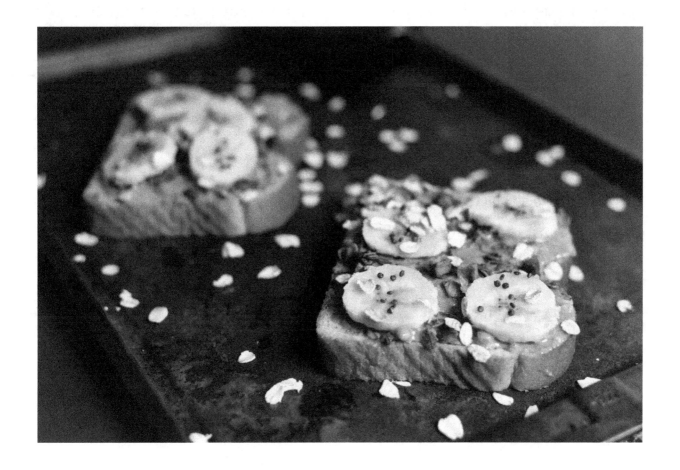

OATMEAL BANANA BOWL

If you're looking for a quick, easy and super nutritious breakfast or snack recipe, this delicious oatmeal bowl is for you. It's ready in just 5 minutes!

MAKES 1 SERVING/ TOTAL TIME 5 MINUTE

INGREDIENTS

3 tbsp instant oats, use gluten-free if needed

1/4 cup or 4 tbsp boiling water

1 banana

1 dragon fruit, see notes

1/4 cup or 4 tbsp plant milk of your choice, we used soy milk

1 tbsp coconut yogurt

METHOD

STEP 1

Add oats and boiling water to a bowl, stir and let stand for 2 to 3 minutes. In the meanwhile, peel and chop the fruit. Add the milk, coconut yogurt and chopped fruit, stir and enjoy your oatmeal bowl.

STEP 2

We used unsweetened soy milk, but feel free to use any sweetened plant milk you want or any sweetener you have on hand.

Best when fresh, keep leftovers in a sealed container in the fridge for 1 to 2 days.

NUTRITION VALUE

254 KJ Energy, 4.8g fat, 0.4g saturated fat, 4.3g fiber, 5.8g protein, 49.9g carbs.

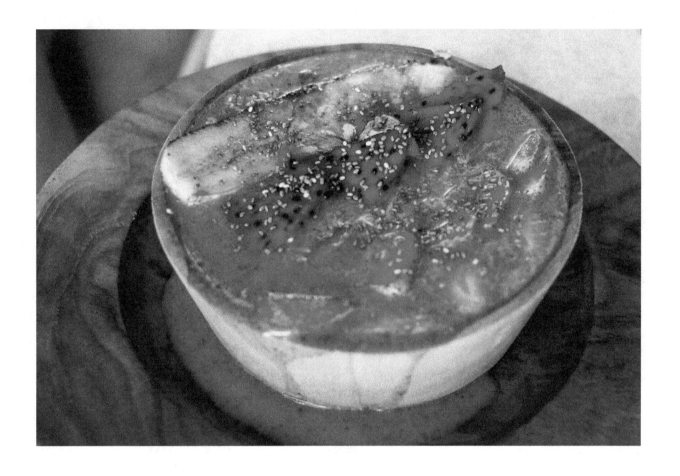

VEGAN WALNUTS GRANOLA

This is a raw version of granola, made with just 5 ingredients in less than 5 minutes. It's a super healthy breakfast or snack recipe!

MAKES 4 SERVING/ TOTAL TIME 5 MINUTE

INGREDIENTS

1 cup walnuts (90 g)

6 Medjool dates, pitted

1/2 cup oats (50 g), gluten-free if needed

2 tbsp ground flax seeds

1/2 tsp cinnamon powder

METHOD

STEP 1

Add the walnuts to a food processor and blend until they have a crumbly texture.

Add the dates and blend again.

Finally, add the rest of the ingredients and blend until well combined.

STEP 2

We served our granola with some banana slices and some soy milk, but you can enjoy it as is, with any plant milk, yogurt, fruit or any ingredient you want.

Keep leftovers in a sealed container at room temperature for 2 to 3 weeks or in the fridge for 3 to 4 weeks.

NUTRITION VALUE	152 KJ Energy, 7.8g fat, 0.5g saturated fat, 3.1g fiber, 4.5g protein, 18.6g carbs.

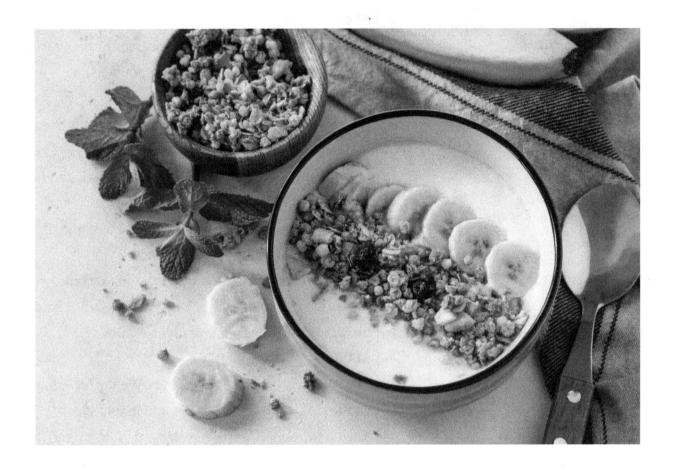

VEGAN BLUEBERRY WAFFLES

Vegan gluten-free blueberry waffles, made with just 5 ingredients in about 30 minutes. Perfect for breakfast served with extra blueberries and maple syrup.

MAKES 5 SERVING/ TOTAL TIME 30 MINUTE

INGREDIENTS

2 and 1/2 cups rolled oats (250 g), use gluten-free if needed

1 and 1/2 cups plant milk of your choice (375 ml), we used oat milk

1/4 cup maple or agave syrup (4 tbsp)

2 tbsp flax seeds

1/2 cup fresh blueberries (80 g)

METHOD

STEP 1

Add the rolled oats to a food processor or blender and pulse until they are ground into a powder-like consistency.

Add the rest of the ingredients (except the blueberries) and pulse again until well combined.

Transfer the batter into a large mixing bowl, add the blueberries and stir until well combined.

Preheat the waffle maker according to manufacturer's directions and add some oil if needed.

Pour the batter into the waffle maker and cook according to manufacturer's instructions until golden brown. Our waffles were ready in 7 minutes.

STEP 2

Serve with your favorite toppings. We topped our waffles with extra blueberries and maple syrup.

Keep leftover waffles in a sealed container in the fridge for about 3 days or in the freezer for 1 month.

NUTRITION VALUE

205 Energy, 4.1g fat, 0.6g saturated fat, 4.7g fiber, 4.9g protein, 37g carbs.

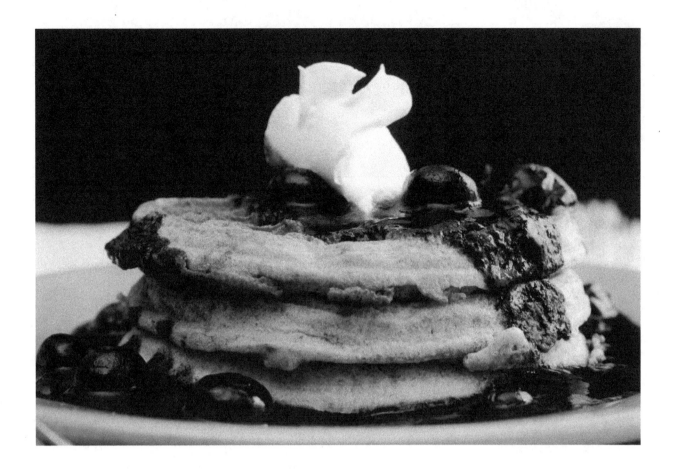

VEGAN PANCAKES

Vegan pancakes, made in less than 20 minutes with 8 simple ingredients. They're so light and fluffy, easy to make, and perfect for breakfast.

MAKES 6 SERVING/ TOTAL TIME 20 MINUTE

INGREDIENTS

1 cup whole wheat flour (120 g)

2 tbsp brown, cane or coconut sugar

2 tsp baking powder

1/4 tsp salt

3/4 cup unsweetened plant milk of your choice (190 ml), I used soy milk

1 flax egg

1 tbsp oil (optional), I used melted coconut oil

1 tsp vanilla extract (optional)

METHOD

STEP 1

Mix dry ingredients in a large bowl (flour, sugar, baking powder, and salt).

Add the liquid ingredients (milk, flax egg, oil, and vanilla extract) to the bowl and stir until well combined. Let the batter stand for 5-10 minutes before using it.

STEP 2

Place 1/4 cup of the batter (65 ml) in a lightly greased hot pan or griddle and cook for about 2 minutes for each side or until golden brown. When the underside is golden and bubbles begin to appear on the surface, it's time to flip over onto the other side. If you don't eat oil, don't grease the pan or griddle, just use a non-stick one. Serve immediately with vegan butter, vegan Nutella, or even raspberry jam. You can also eat them with maple syrup, cacao nibs, and fresh fruit, or serve them with your favorite plant milk.

NUTRITION VALUE

124 KJ Energy, 3.7g fat, 2.4g saturated fat, 3.1g fiber, 3.9g protein, 20.2g carbs.

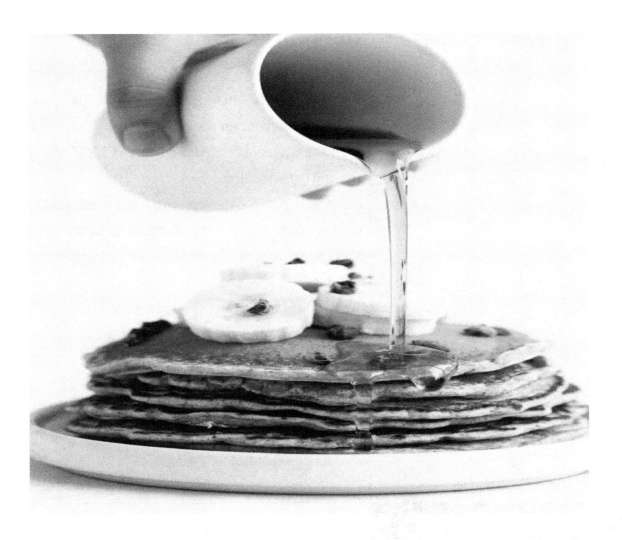

BERRY AND ORANGE COMPOTE

Berry compote, sweet, fruity, and delicious. It's nutritious, it requires only 4 ingredients and it's ready in just 15 minutes.

MAKES 4 SERVING/ TOTAL TIME 20 MINUTE

INGREDIENTS

1 cup strawberries (150 g), chopped

1 cup blueberries (150 g)

2 tbsp orange juice

METHOD

STEP 1

Put all the ingredients together in a saucepan and cook over medium heat until it boils.

After that, cook over medium heat for 10-15 minutes, stirring occasionally.

If the fruit is already sweet, you don't need to add any kind of sweetener, but you might want to try it and add some sugar to taste if you'd like your compote sweeter.

STEP 2

Serve your favorite sweet dishes with this vegan compote for a delicious fruity taste.

Keep the leftovers in a sealed container for 7-10 days or in the freezer for up to 1 month.

NUTRITION VALUE

24 KJ Energy, 0.2g fat, 1.1g fiber, 0.4g protein, 5.9g carbs.

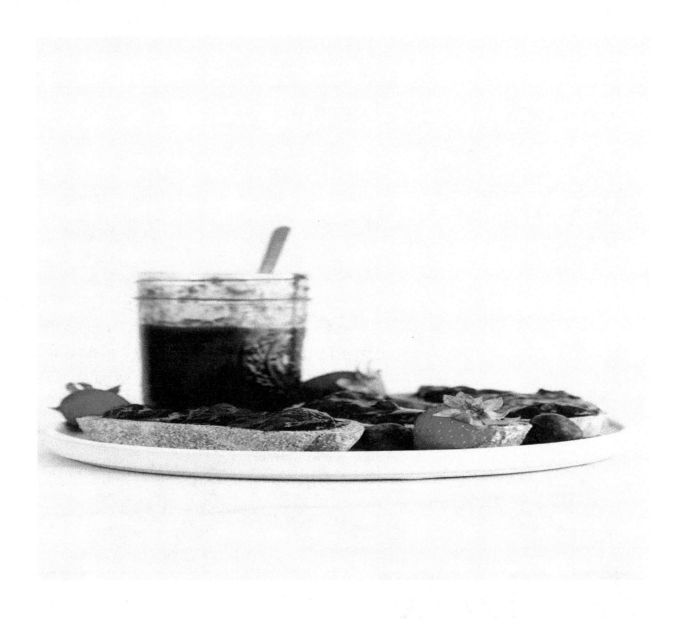

COCONUT CREAMY

Coconut butter, a creamy, tasty, and delightful recipe It's extremely easy to make and it only requires 1 ingredient and 2 minutes of your time!

MAKES 1 SERVING/ TOTAL TIME 2 MINUTE

INGREDIENTS

3 cups shredded or desiccated unsweetened coconut (270 g)

METHOD

STEP 1

Add the shredded coconut to a blender or food processor and blend until smooth.

STEP 2

Serve with some raspberry jam toasts, in smoothies like a mango smoothie, or add it to your morning oatmeal. It would also taste great on some baked sweet potatoes or squash or as a replacement for cashew butter (or any other kind of vegan butter) in any recipe.

Keep the leftovers in an airtight container in the fridge for at least 2 weeks.

NUTRITION VALUE

60 KJ Energy, 5.6g fat, 5g saturated fat, 1.5g fiber, 0.6g protein, 2.6g carbs.

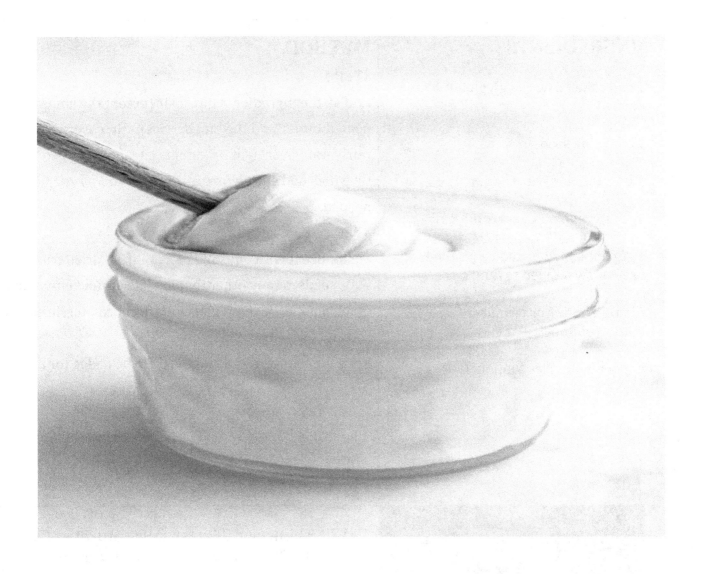

CHIA OVERNIGHT OATS

Overnight oats, a delicious, healthy, and nutritious breakfast or snack. It's ready in just 10 minutes with only 7 ingredients, and great to eat on the go!

MAKES 2 SERVING/ TOTAL TIME 10 MINUTE

INGREDIENTS

1 cup rolled oats (90 g), gluten-free if needed

1 tbsp chia seeds

1 tbsp maple syrup (optional)

1/2 tsp vanilla extract (optional)

1 cup milk of your choice (250 ml), I used unsweetened soy milk

Almond butter or peanut butter (optional)

Fresh blueberries (optional)

METHOD

STEP 1

Add all the ingredients into a jar (except the almond or peanut butter and the blueberries), stir, cover, and refrigerate overnight or for at least 4 hours.

Give it a good stir before serving and add more milk if needed.

STEP 2

Customize it with any kind of fresh fruit, dried fruits, nuts, seeds, or any other topping like ground cinnamon, cocoa powder, ground ginger, dark chocolate, shredded coconut, or matcha tea.

Keep the leftovers in a closed jar in the fridge for up to 3-4 days.

NUTRITION VALUE

177 KJ Energy, 7.2g fat, 0.9g saturated fat, 6.1g fiber, 8.3g protein, 19.9g carbs.

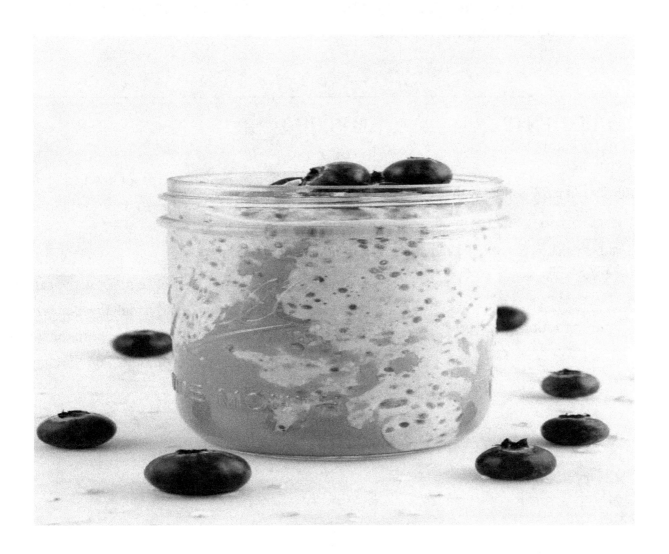

ECHINACEA AND CARROTS JUICE

Ward off cold and flu viruses by drinking this mixture of vegetable juice and echinacea tea daily- the vegies contain anti-oxidants and vitamin C, while echinacea boosts immune function.

MAKES 2 SERVING/ TOTAL TIME 15 MINUTE

INGREDIENTS

1 echinacea tea bag

80ml (1/3 cup) boiling water

2 large carrots, peeled, topped

1 red capsicum, halved, deseeded, thickly sliced

1 lime, peeled

Ice cubes (optional), to serve

METHOD

STEP 1

Place the tea bag in a small heatproof bowl and pour over boiling water. Set aside for 10 minutes to infuse.

STEP 2

Meanwhile, use a juice extractor to process the carrot, capsicum and lime. Transfer to a small jug. Squeeze all the liquid from the tea bag. Pour the tea into the jug. Add the ice cubes and stir to combine. Pour among glasses to serve.

NUTRITION VALUE

265 KJ Energy, 0.5g fat, 6g fiber, 3g protein, 12g carbs.

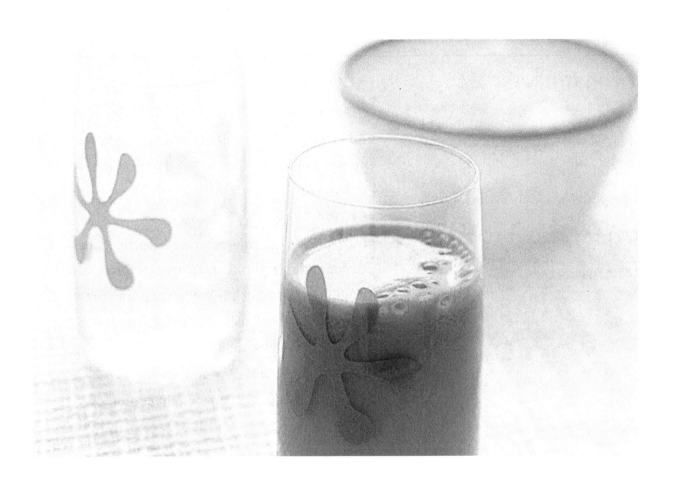

CHIA MAPLE SYRUP PUDDING

Chia pudding, a delicious breakfast, snack, or dessert, made in just 5 minutes with only 4 ingredients. It's sweet, creamy, healthy, and nutritious!

MAKES 2 SERVING/ TOTAL TIME 5 MINUTE

INGREDIENTS

2 cups unsweetened plant milk of your choice (500 ml), I used homemade coconut milk

2 tbsp maple syrup

1/2 tsp vanilla extract (optional)

1/2 cup chia seeds (85 g)

METHOD

STEP 1

Add the liquid ingredients to a mixing bowl (plant milk, syrup, and vanilla extract) and whisk until well combined.

STEP 2

Incorporate the chia seeds and whisk again.

Cover and refrigerate overnight or for at least 2 hours.

When ready to eat, stir well, serve, and top with ingredients like fresh fruit, dried fruit, nuts, seeds, cacao nibs, dark chocolate, jam... Or even with a little bit of coconut butter or almond butter!

Keep the leftovers in an airtight container in the fridge for 4-5 days.

NUTRITION VALUE

157 KJ Energy, 6.7 fat, 0.7g saturated fat, 11.7g fiber, 5g protein, 20.5g carbs.

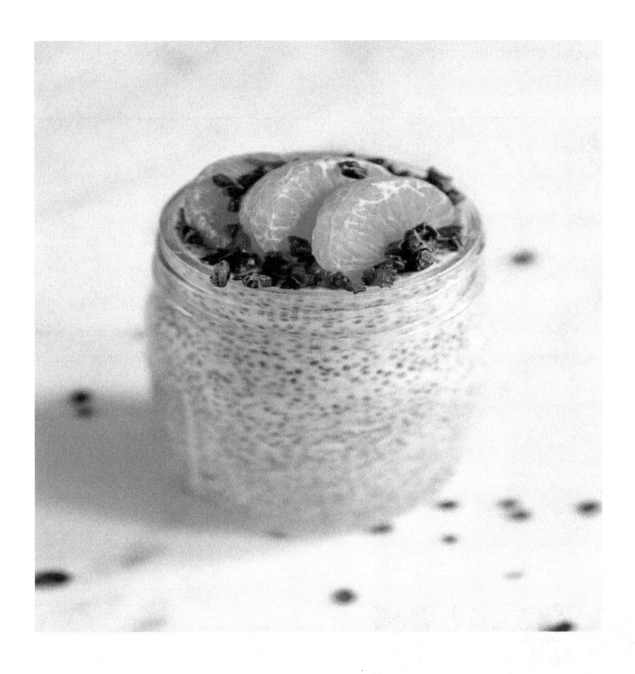

TROPICAL FRUIT SALAD

Recipe that everyone loves!

MAKES 6 SERVING/ TOTAL TIME 2 HOUR 20 MINUTE

INGREDIENTS

1 pineapple, peeled, chopped

2 mangoes, peeled, chopped

3 kiwifruits, peeled, chopped

2 bananas, peeled, chopped

1 bunch black grapes

8 fresh or canned lychees

3 passion fruit, halved, pulp removed

METHOD

STEP 1

Combine pineapple, mangoes, kiwifruit, bananas and grapes in a large bowl.

STEP 2

Peel and discard skins and seeds from lychees (if fresh). Add to fruit salad with passion fruit pulp. Toss gently to combine. Cover. Refrigerate for 2 hours or until chilled. Serve.

NUTRITION VALUE

737 KJ Energy, 1g fat,
8g fiber, 3g protein, 36g carbs.

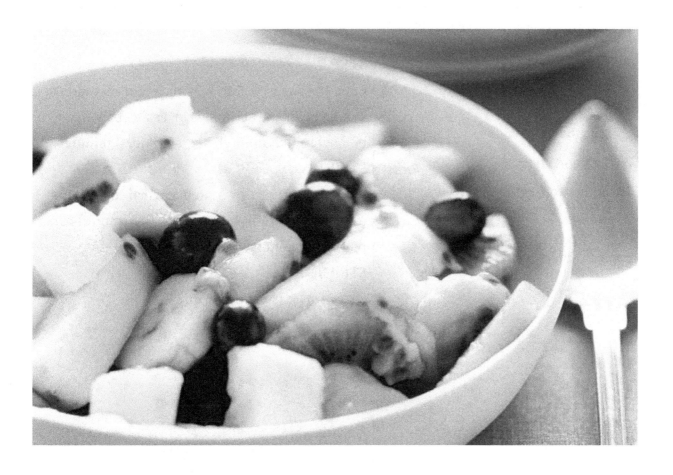

POACHED DRIED FRUITS

Recipe that everyone loves!

MAKES 4 SERVING/ TOTAL TIME 55 MINUTE

INGREDIENTS

1/2 cup brown sugar

1 1/2 cups water

grated rind of 1 lemon

2 cinnamon sticks

1 vanilla bean, split lengthways, scraped (see note)

400g dried fruit salad (apricots, prunes, apples, pears)

METHOD

STEP 1

Combine sugar, water, lemon rind, cinnamon sticks, and vanilla bean and scrapings in a saucepan. Bring to the boil over medium-high heat. Boil for 3 minutes.

STEP 2

Add dried fruits. Cover. Reduce heat to low. Cook for 40 to 45 minutes, stirring occasionally, or until fruit is plump and tender.

STEP 3

Serve warm fruits in syrup.

NUTRITION VALUE

1555 KJ Energy, 1g fat, 6g fiber, 2g protein, 85g carbs.

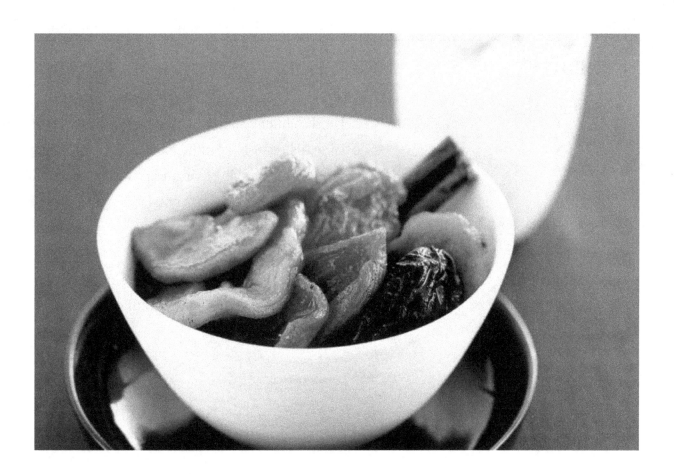

VEGAN COOKBOOK BREAKFAST EDITION- DANA TAYLOR

GINGER INFUSED FRUIT SALAD

A hint of ginger adds an extra dimension to this juicy fruit salad.

MAKES 4 SERVING/ TOTAL TIME 60 MINUTE

INGREDIENTS

3 mandarins

2 Ruby grapefruit

2 oranges

2 tangelos

2 tablespoons caster sugar

1 teaspoon finely grated fresh ginger

METHOD

STEP 1

Peel and segment mandarins, removing as much pith as possible. Using a sharp knife, peel grapefruit, oranges and tangelos, removing skin and pith. Segment fruit between membranes over a bowl, reserving juice. Place fruit segments into bowl.

STEP 2

Sprinkle fruit with sugar and ginger. Gently toss to combine. Cover and refrigerate until chilled. Spoon into glasses. Serve.

NUTRITION VALUE

667 KJ Energy, 1g fat,
6g fiber, 3g protein, 32g carbs.

94

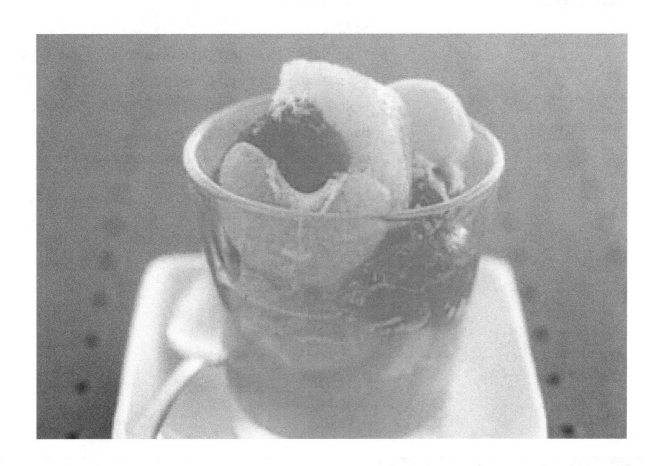

SHOOTING FRUIT SKEWERS

Let the kids make a point with these fruity skewers. They're easy to make and even easier to eat!

MAKES 4 SERVING/ TOTAL TIME 15 MINUTE

INGREDIENTS

1 (1.5kg) honeydew melon

2 large bananas

1 tablespoon orange juice

8 strawberries, hulled

METHOD

STEP 1

Trim ends from melon. Cut crossways into 1cm-thick slices. Using a 4cm star-shaped cutter, cut 12 stars from melon. Set aside. Peel bananas. Trim ends. Cut each banana crossways into quarters. Place in a bowl. Drizzle with orange juice. Toss gently to coat.

STEP 2

Thread honeydew stars, strawberries and banana on skewers. Serve.

NUTRITION VALUE

814 KJ Energy, 1g fat,
5g fiber, 4g protein, 39g carbs.

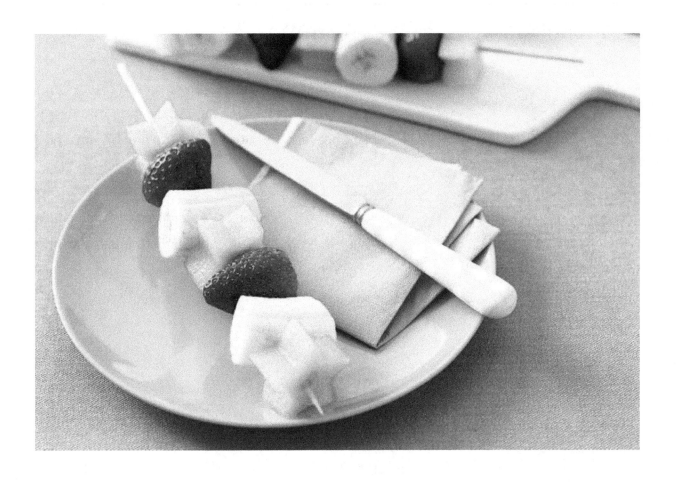

FRUITS MARINATED

You can use any seasonal fruit of your choice in this recipe - strawberries, figs and mango all work well.

MAKES 6 SERVING/ TOTAL TIME 40 MINUTE

INGREDIENTS

3/4 cup (165g) caster sugar

1 vanilla bean, split, seeds scraped

2-3 tablespoons or brandy or kirsch (optional)

2-3 peaches, thinly sliced

3 cup berries

4 small nectarines, peeled

1 orange, peeled, segmented

1 cup cherries

1 punnet (150g) blueberries

1 punnet (150g) raspberries

METHOD
STEP 1
Place sugar in a saucepan with 1 cup (250ml) water and vanilla. Stir over low heat until sugar is dissolved; simmer for 5 minutes, then cool. Add brandy, if using.

STEP 2
Layer the fruits in a large sterilized jar, then pour the cooled syrup over top. Seal and store in fridge before transporting.

NUTRITION VALUE

1042 KJ Energy,
7g fiber, 3g protein, 32.2g carbs.

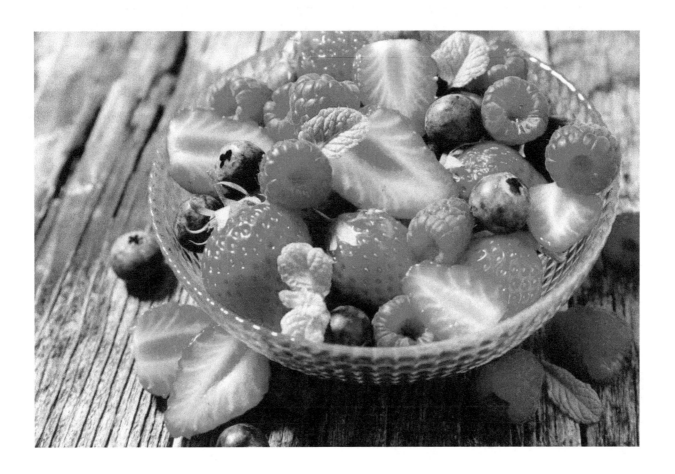

WATERMELON GINGER GRANITA

Recipe that everyone loves!

MAKES 4 SERVING/ TOTAL TIME 10 MINUTE

INGREDIENTS

1kg piece seedless watermelon, skin removed, cut into chunks

2 cups ice cubes

1/4 cup fresh mint leaves

2 tablespoons caster sugar

1 teaspoon finely grated fresh ginger

METHOD

STEP 1

Place watermelon in a blender. Blend until finely chopped. Add ice, mint leaves, sugar and ginger. Blend until ice is crushed.

STEP 2

Pour into serving glasses and serve immediately.

NUTRITION VALUE

475 KJ Energy, 1g fat, 2g fiber, 1g protein, 24g carbs.

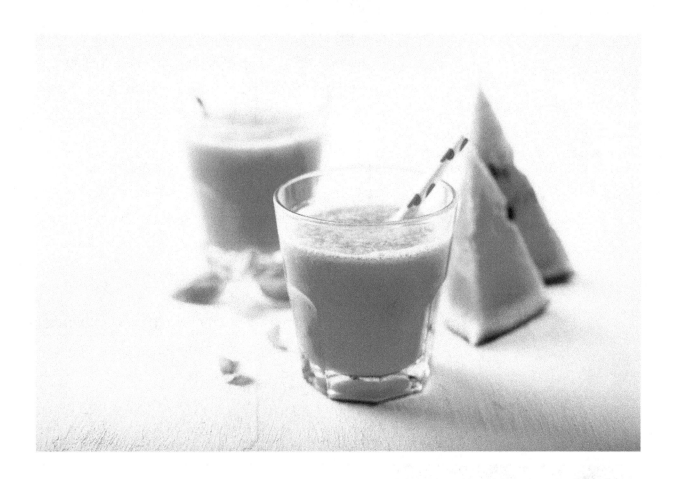

WATERMELON LIME GRANITA

This watermelon and lime frozen granite is a crowd-pleaser.

MAKES 6 SERVING/ TOTAL TIME 9 HOUR 40 MINUTE

INGREDIENTS

1 cup water

2 to 3 limes, juiced

3/4 cup white sugar

1/4 (1kg) seedless watermelon, peeled, cut into pieces, deseeded

METHOD

STEP 1

Heat water, 1/3 cup of juice and sugar in a saucepan over low heat, stirring, until sugar dissolves. Add melon. Bring to the boil. Reduce heat. Simmer for 3 minutes.

STEP 2

Process one-third of mixture in a food processor until smooth. Pour into a 3cm deep, 30cm x 20cm lamington pan. Process remaining mixture in 2 batches. Transfer to pan. Cool completely. Cover. Freeze for 8 hours or until set.

STEP 3

Remove from freezer. Stand for 10 to 20 minutes, or until soft enough to run a fork through. Spoon into glasses. Serve.

NUTRITION VALUE

684 KJ Energy, 1g fat,
2g fiber, 1g protein, 37g carbs.

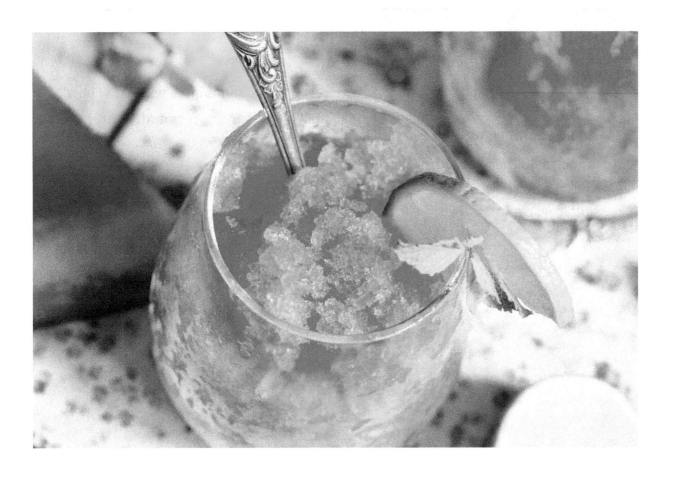

PASSION FRUIT AND SUGAR MINT

Delicious mouthfuls with an extra zing.

MAKES 4 SERVING/ TOTAL TIME 20 MINUTE

INGREDIENTS

1 1/2 cups caster sugar

1 cup of mint leaves, roughly chopped

1 small pineapple, cut into long pieces

1 small rock melon, de-seeded, peeled and cut into long pieces

4 passion fruit, cut into halves

METHOD

STEP 1

Place caster sugar and mint leaves in the bowl of a small food processor. Process until mint is finely chopped.

STEP 2

Place the mint sugar into a serving bowl and serve with fresh fruit pieces. The fruit can be "dipped" into the mint sugar or served sprinkled with mint sugar.

NUTRITION VALUE

1707 KJ Energy,
6 fiber, 2g protein, 95g carbs.

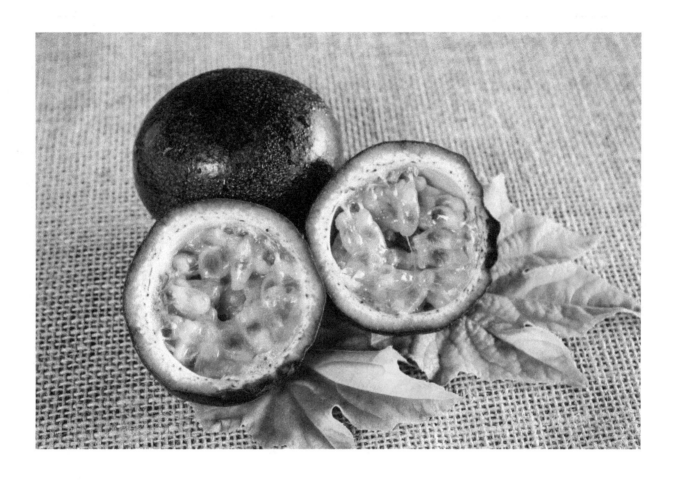

PINEAPPLE LYCHEES SALAD

Recipe that everyone loves!

MAKES 4 SERVING/ TOTAL TIME 20 MINUTE

INGREDIENTS

850g pineapple, thin wedges

400g can lychees, drained

GINGER DRESSING

1 cup sugar

1 1/2 cups water

50g ginger, sliced

METHOD

STEP 1

Place sugar in a saucepan with water and ginger. Stir over medium heat until sugar has dissolved, then increase heat. Simmer for 6-7 minutes or until reduced slightly and thickened. Remove from heat, reserving some of the ginger strips, and cool.

STEP 2

Toss pineapple with lychees and pour over ginger syrup. Garnish with reserved ginger strips.

NUTRITION VALUE

1431KJ Energy, 1g fat,
5g fiber, 2g protein, 79g carbs.

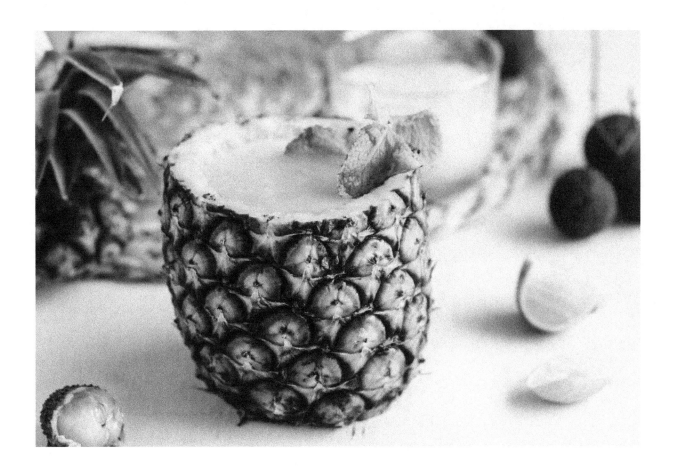

CPSIA information can be obtained
at www.ICGtesting.com
Printed in the USA
BVHW011643120521
606944BV00020B/2024